MAKING SENSE OF CHRONIC PAIN

How it works, why it lingers, and what you can do about it.

by Jerry Curry

Broken Script Press

© 2025 Broken Script Press
All rights reserved.

No part of this book may be reproduced, stored in a retrieval system, or transmitted in any form or by any means—electronic, mechanical, photocopying, recording, or otherwise—without prior written permission of the publisher, except for brief quotations used in reviews or critical articles.

Published by Broken Script Press
www.Brokenscriptpress.com

DISCLAIMER

This book is for educational and informational purposes only. It is not intended to diagnose, treat, cure, or prevent any medical condition. Nothing in these pages should be taken as medical advice or as a substitute for consultation with a licensed healthcare professional.

Every person's body, medical history, and pain experience is different. Always talk with your physician or qualified healthcare provider about any questions you have regarding a medical condition, symptoms, or treatment options. Never delay seeking professional care because of something you have read in this book.

The author and publisher disclaim all liability for any actions taken or not taken based on the material presented here.

Table of Contents

Introduction 6

You're Not Crazy 6

Pain Maps 17

Why Pain Persists 39

The Emotional Brain 65

Fibromyalgia 99

Ehlers Danlos Syndrome 137

Other Conditions That Hijack the Pain System 169

Why This Lens Matters 197

Movement As Medicine 217

Sleep, Safety, and Foundations of Rest 241

Recovery Tools 267

Rebuilding Trust in Your Body 297

Living in a World That Does Not Understand 319

Building Your Own Map Forward 345

Glossary of Terms 379

Recommended Reading 418

Master Bibliography 426

About the Author 462

Introduction

You're Not Crazy

If you're reading this, you've likely been experiencing pain for a long time.

You may have bounced from doctor to doctor, getting test after test run to show no results. You've likely tried numerous therapists who offer every treatment available. Each one promised answers. Few delivered lasting change. Maybe you've been handed vague diagnoses or told everything looks "normal." Perhaps you've been told, or slowly started to believe, that it's all in your head. And maybe, like so many others, you're tired. Not just from the pain itself, but from the constant effort it takes to convince people that it's real.

You're not alone. And you're not crazy.

What you're experiencing is real. But it may not be what you think it is. This book is built on a simple but powerful premise. Chronic pain isn't just about damaged tissue. It's about the way your nervous system has learned to perceive threat. And if it can be learned, it can be unlearned.

You might feel like you're losing your mind, because how else are you supposed to make sense of all this? One day, your hip aches. Another day, it's your shoulder. Then your hands tingle, or your skin burns for no reason you can find. You may wake up feeling like you never slept. You try to describe it to your doctor, and his response leaves you feeling dismissed. You try to explain it to your partner, and they tell you maybe you need to hit the gym more… or suck it up. Sometimes you feel as though the words don't land. They make sense to you, but no one seems to hear them. You catch the looks, the polite nods, the way people drift off mid-sentence. They don't get it, and a part of you starts to wonder if they ever will.

You've tried everything you could think of. You've explored all the internet "gurus" preaching about diets and supplements. You've rested, exercised, journaled, and tracked every symptom. You've read more medical blogs than most med students. And still, no clear answers. Just more questions. More confusion.

Sometimes, you're not even sure you believe yourself anymore.

That's the moment something shifts. Not just in your body, but in your sense of self. When it stops being about pain and starts to feel like you're disappearing under it.

Chronic pain affects millions of people from all walks of life. According to the CDC, more than 50 million adults in the United States live with some form of chronic pain.[1] It's one of the leading causes of disability, lost work, and rising healthcare costs. And yet, for something so common, it's still profoundly misunderstood.

For many people, pain starts with a real injury or condition. However, what's often overlooked is that pain doesn't always subside when the injury heals. In fact, that's usually when things become more confusing and isolating.

You're not broken. You're not imagining it. But the map you were given to understand your body and your pain? That map is incomplete. And no one gave you a manual.

I've seen the same patterns emerge again and again in over 2 decades of working with chronic pain. I've worked with athletes, office workers, as well as stay-at-home parents. I've worked with individuals in their 20s, and those in their 70s: people with different lives and diagnoses. But the same core pattern always emerges. A nervous system that learned to protect in ways that no longer serve. That's what this book is about. Not the diagnosis. But the pattern beneath it.

Someone develops pain that doesn't fit neatly into traditional medical boxes. And because the system doesn't know what to do with them, it minimizes, dismisses, or pathologizes their experience. Over time, that confusion starts to erode trust, not just in the system, but in themselves.

By the time they walk into my practice, they're often exhausted, over-informed, and quietly hoping that this time will be different. Some have already given up. Some have fused their identity to the pain because it's the only constant. Others are hanging on by a thread, wanting to move forward but unsure how.

Look, I'm not going to pretend to understand what you're going through here. I don't know what it's like to have your body speak a language that no one else seems to recognize. But I do know what it feels like to be dismissed. To be told your experience doesn't make sense. To be speaking, yet feel unheard.

I don't have all the answers. And I'm skeptical of anyone who claims they do. But I've spent decades searching for a better way to understand pain, especially the kind that makes people feel like strangers in their own bodies. The sort of pain that doesn't follow the rules and resists explanation. Pain that isn't just physical, but personal, isolating, disorienting. That kind of pain has been my focus, and finding what actually helps has been my life's work.

I won't promise you a miracle cure. I won't hand you a rigid protocol or tell you that if you believe hard enough, the pain will vanish. What I will offer is a different way to understand what's happening, and a framework for working with it. That's no less powerful. And it's more honest.

Modern research has demonstrated that the nervous system can "learn" to perceive pain in a manner similar to how it acquires a skill. Scientists refer to this phenomenon as maladaptive neuroplasticity, the brain's ability to rewire itself in ways that reinforce pain signals even when no injury remains.[2] In the chapters ahead, we'll explore how this happens and, more importantly, how someone can change it.

Numerous books are available on chronic pain. Some focus on biology. Others focus on psychology. A few give protocols or exercises. However, most overlook the connection between the two: how your nervous system learns about pain and how that learning influences everything from your movement to your mood and sense of identity.

This book bridges that gap. It isn't just about understanding pain. It's about understanding your pain and why it's been so difficult to change.

This book isn't going to tell you to push through pain or just relax. It also won't allow you to blame yourself for not getting better. But it will ask you to consider that your pain is not a life sentence. It's a signal your nervous system learned to send. And as anything learned, it can be unlearned. You're not broken. You're caught in a loop. This book will help you identify the edges of that loop, allowing you to begin stepping out of it.

Before we go further, I want to be clear about something. This book is not intended to be used as ammunition against your doctor, physical therapist, or any other healthcare practitioner. The vast majority of these professionals exist to help you. And most healthcare providers genuinely care and are doing their best within a system that wasn't designed to explain or treat pain like yours. What this book offers is a better framework, one that can help you have more productive conversations with your care team. It's about giving you language to help them see what they might be missing. Ideally, it opens their minds to seeing your pain through a different lens. At the very least, it can act as a filter, helping you decide whether a practitioner is a good fit for you. The goal isn't to dismiss professional care. It's to help you engage with it more effectively.

You'll learn how pain becomes a pattern. You'll notice how that pattern manifests in your daily life. You'll understand why some treatments may have failed, not because they were useless, but because they didn't address the whole picture. And you'll start to see where your influence lies, and how to take the next step from there.

A quick note on the writing style of this book: I've done my best to avoid making it feel like a textbook. That said, we'll need to discuss brain anatomy and nervous system function to make the case for how pain works. Don't worry, I've worked hard to make those explanations as clear and accessible as possible. You don't need to memorize names or draw diagrams. You just need to understand that multiple systems are at play and how they interact. Later in the book, I'll remind you of this again. You don't need to remember every structure or term. You only need to see the pattern.

In Part I, we'll explore how pain works, not just in theory, but in your body. In Part II, we'll look at specific conditions like Fibromyalgia, Ehlers-Danlos Syndrome, CRPS, and PTSD, as well as a few others, and how, in some ways, they all stem from the same root system. These aren't just separate diseases with separate causes. They're different expressions of the same underlying dysfunction. Your nervous system has become stuck in a threat response. These conditions are complex, and this isn't an attempt to minimize them or the mechanics behind them. Understanding this doesn't minimize your diagnosis. Instead, it reframes it in a way that makes change possible.

In Part III, we'll talk about what you can actually do with this knowledge. I won't give you rigid protocols, but I'll offer adaptable principles you can make your own. There won't be a 30-day challenge or a step-by-step cure. What you will find are principles that are backed by research and refined through practice. Some of those will resonate immediately; others might take time. The goal isn't perfection, it's finding what works for your nervous system, and at your pace.

Maybe you've been dismissed, gaslit, or told your pain is "just stress." Suppose you are one of those who have tried everything and are tired of being told to try harder. You may be beginning to lose faith in your own body and want to find a way back to trust, even if the pain never entirely goes away. If any or all of this describes you, then this book is for you.

This book is *not* for those seeking a quick fix, a miracle supplement, or a guide to tell them exactly what to do at every step. It's not for those who want to be told their pain is purely physical and will disappear with the right injection or surgery. And it's not for people who aren't ready to consider that their nervous system plays a role in their experience. If that's you, that's okay. But this book probably isn't the right fit.

It doesn't matter whether it's labeled as Fibromyalgia, Ehlers-Danlos Syndrome, autoimmune pain, long-standing injuries, or something your doctors haven't even named. The principles we'll cover here apply across the board. Yes, your experience of pain is unique, and that uniqueness matters. But beneath all those differences lies a shared root. Pain is a signal, and it can become altered, exaggerated, or stuck in a loop even when it appears differently to each person. Recognizing that common thread doesn't diminish your experience, it helps explain it. And it opens the door to change.

What's required is a new lens and a different kind of conversation.

The point of this isn't to lecture you. It's a conversation. I'll share insights from science, from the treatment room, and from the people who've trusted me to walk with them through their pain.

If nothing has worked for you yet, that's okay. It doesn't mean you've failed. It means that nothing has been able to fully explain what is actually happening. And that means there's still room for something new.

You don't need to believe in quick fixes. You need to know that your system can learn, and that you can be part of that process. This isn't about willpower or positive thinking. You didn't think yourself into this, and you won't think yourself out of it. What you can do is provide your nervous system with new information consistently, over time. That's not the same as "trying harder." It's about working *with* your system, not against it.

This book will help you ask better questions, communicate more clearly with your healthcare providers, and reconnect with your body in ways that foster strength, resilience, and confidence, rather than fear.

You don't need perfect. You need a new starting point.

If you're still searching for a way forward, one that respects your pain but doesn't let it define you, you're in the right place.

Let's begin.

Endnotes

[1] Dahlhamer, J., Lucas, J., Zelaya, C., et al. (2018). Prevalence of chronic pain and high-impact chronic pain among adults — United States, 2016. *Morbidity and Mortality Weekly Report*, 67(36), 1001–1006.

[2] Moseley, G. L., & Butler, D. S. (2015). Fifteen years of explaining pain: The past, present, and future. *Journal of Pain*, 16(9), 807–813.

Chapter 1

Pain Maps

I wasn't always on board with this way of thinking.

In my first year of practice, I was working in a clinic when a patient broke down in front of me. She'd been dismissed by countless providers before me, seen as too emotional and too complicated. We were wrapping up our session, and she was crying, saying she had a headache at the base of her skull.

I didn't know what to do. I had another patient waiting, and I was already behind schedule. All I could think to do was gently rest my hand on the back of her head, where she said it hurt. I held it there for maybe 30 seconds.

She stopped crying. Looked at me. "Oh," she said. "My headache's gone. Thank you."

I told her she was welcome, but I couldn't help thinking, "Lady, you're crazy."

That moment stuck with me. I couldn't explain what had just happened, so I dismissed it. When something doesn't align with the framework we've been taught, our instinct is to brush it off and keep moving. I had been taught that trigger points followed predictable patterns, and that referred pain had to match anatomical logic. There was no nerve linking the base of her skull to her emotional trauma, no chart that could explain why simply being touched could bring her pain down.

The more patients I saw, the more I realized that the old model was no longer effective. It's not as though I needed to rebel against it just for the sake of doing so. It simply didn't explain what I was witnessing repeatedly in real people with real pain. Technique and pressure definitely matter when working with tissue. However, I could not ignore the fact that sometimes just being present and giving a specific area attention had just as much, or sometimes even more, impact than anything I had previously been taught. Many times, pain didn't even follow the anatomy charts I'd memorized. And the people labeled "too sensitive" were often the ones working hardest to make sense of it all. Yet, it was something that no one had ever taken the time to explain.

That moment cracked the foundation for me. Questions started to pour in, and I dove deep into concepts like neuroplasticity, the brain's role in pain, and how trauma rewires our internal maps. As for the work I was doing, I didn't stop believing in it, nor did I think it wasn't effective. I saw the results daily. What happened, however, was that I stopped assuming I understood why it was working.

I'd been taught all the mechanisms of how massage and manual therapy worked. Release the fascia, deactivate the trigger point, improve circulation, break up adhesions. But perhaps that understanding was incomplete. What I came to realize was that the tissues and structures I was working with provided me with direct access to the person's nervous system. After all, it was the nervous system that controlled all the structures I was trying to affect. Any change in those tissues wasn't just a local mechanical shift. It was a direct consequence of a change in the nervous system itself.

That woman with the headache? Perhaps resting my hand on her head was enough stimulus to overwrite her pain signal. To create, even if only temporarily, a new signal that didn't include pain. This idea may not add up yet. It may sound far-fetched. But trust me, it will make sense soon. I still think that client often. I hope that after all her dismissals, she finally found the answers she deserved.

Pain That Doesn't Add Up

Pain doesn't always make sense. At least not in the way we are taught to understand it. From an early age, we grow up believing that pain equals damage: that if something hurts, something must be broken. And once it heals, the pain should disappear. But for millions of people living with chronic pain, that equation doesn't add up. The injury is long gone, yet the pain remains, just as real, just as intense.

Sometimes that lingering pain is the result of compensatory movement patterns that developed during an injury but never corrected afterward. At other times, chronic overuse, poor posture, or muscular imbalances can result in constant strain on the tissues. Or in most cases, a combination of all three. Sometimes, it's the underlying muscle weakness that sets those faulty patterns in motion. In others, it's the injury itself that triggers faulty movement, which then becomes the new norm. Pain can be reinforced by this even after the tissue has healed. Even these faulty patterns are messages, but they aren't just sent to the brain. The brain establishes them as part of a loop.

Once a pain signal is repeated enough, the brain starts to expect it, reinforcing a faulty pattern that becomes part of how it perceives and manages the body. Sometimes the injury never fully heals. But for many, the real issue is how the nervous system has adapted to the pain, not just the initial damage that triggered it.

A typical example is low back pain. Someone might strain their back shoveling snow. The tissue heals in a matter of weeks, but the pain persists. Why? Because the nervous system has "learned" that pain response. Each time it repeats, the path becomes more deeply carved into the system. The brain continues to send out warnings long after the original threat is gone. We will explore this concept more in the second chapter.

The same thing can happen with a shoulder injury that heals but later manifests as elbow or neck pain, or after knee surgery, when the pain spreads to the hip. When pain lingers, it's not a matter of weakness of will. It's your brain and body reinforcing pathways that have become second nature.

So what's actually happening? What if pain sticks around long after the injury is gone? What if scans look normal, but the pain is still real? What if different doctors give you different explanations, or worse, none at all? That's when you start to question not just your body, but your sanity.

Pain is a real phenomenon. However, what's often overlooked is why it's real and how your brain has learned to interpret it. These strange lingering pains aren't random. They actually reflect the brain's ability to adapt, sometimes with unintended consequences. But for us to understand why this happens, we need to look at what the brain is actually doing. That's where the story really begins.

Maladaptive Neuroplasticity: A Brief Introduction

To make sense of what's really happening in chronic pain, we have to talk about something called maladaptive neuroplasticity. Maladaptive neuroplasticity simply means the brain has adapted in a way that works against you rather than for you. The term grew out of neuroscience research in the late 1990s and early 2000s, when scientists discovered that the brain's learning mechanisms can just as easily reinforce pain and protective patterns as they can reinforce healthy ones. It's widely used in clinical and scientific fields, including neurology, physical therapy, and pain research. This is a key thread running through almost every persistent pain condition. It doesn't matter if the original cause of it was an injury, emotional trauma, repetitive strain, poor posture, or just stress. The real issue often lies in how your brain and nervous system have adapted to these changes.

Neuroplasticity refers to the brain's ability to learn and adapt in response to experience. It's how we grow, recover, and develop new skills. But sometimes that same learning system works against us. When pain signals are sent repeatedly, the brain begins to reinforce those pathways. Pain becomes wired in, not imagined, not exaggerated, but learned.[1]

This is why phantom limb pain happens. A person can feel pain in a limb that isn't there because the brain's map for that limb continues to fire.[2] Or why someone might strain their back shoveling snow, heal in a matter of weeks, but continue to experience pain months later. The tissue has healed, but the nervous system has "learned" that pain response. And each time it repeats, the path becomes more deeply carved into the system, and the brain continues to send warnings long after the original threat has passed. A client of mine described this phenomenon perfectly. Years after successfully fighting cancer, she developed COVID. During her illness, she felt the same specific low back pain that she'd experienced during her cancer treatment. But this time, she recognized it for what it was. She told me she remembered thinking, "Wow, look how my body remembered that." The back pain wasn't caused by new damage. It was a learned pattern, reactivated by the familiar context of systemic illness and immune stress. Her nervous system had stored that pain response and replayed it when similar circumstances arose. That's maladaptive neuroplasticity in action. A prime example of the system pulling from its memory bank and producing pain not because something is wrong, but because it recognizes the situation as threatening.

So while many different things can trigger pain, what keeps it going is often the result of these reinforced neural circuits. The nervous system becomes better at producing pain the more it does it. Understanding how this works is the foundation for changing it. However, to get there, we first need to understand the mechanisms at play. How the nervous system actually learns pain. And where exactly in the body and brain this happens. Let's look at the systems involved.

When the System Gets Stuck: Central Sensitization

Central sensitization is one of the most essential concepts in modern pain science, yet it's rarely explained to patients in a way that makes sense. At its core, central sensitization refers to the phenomenon in which the central nervous system becomes more sensitive to stimulation and/or pain signals.[3] It's what happens when the nervous system becomes hypersensitive, amplifying normal or even mild sensations into painful ones.

Imagine a smoke alarm that has been triggered so many times that it now goes off when you toast bread. The alarm isn't broken, exactly. It's just become hypersensitive. That's central sensitization.

Normally, pain signals travel from the body to the spinal cord and then up to the brain. Along the way, these signals are regulated; some are amplified, while others are dampened, depending on the context. However, when pain signals are repeatedly sent, the neurons in the spinal cord and brain begin to change. They become more excitable. Over time, even gentle touch or movement can be perceived as painful.[4]

This process is called "wind-up." With each repeated pain signal, the response intensifies, much like a crescendo that never stops.[5] Eventually, the nervous system reaches a point where it's stuck in high alert, interpreting even normal sensations as threats.

Two key phenomena emerge from central sensitization:

Allodynia – pain from stimuli that are normally non-painful. A light touch, a soft fabric, or even air movement across the skin can feel like a burn or a stab. This happens because the brain has lowered its threshold for what it considers dangerous.[6]

Hyperalgesia – an exaggerated pain response to mildly painful stimuli. A small bump or pressure that would normally cause brief discomfort instead produces intense, prolonged pain.[7]

What's driving this hypersensitivity? Part of it is chemical. Repeated pain signals trigger the release of neurotransmitters such as glutamate and substance P in the spinal cord, which excite neurons and make them more reactive. But there's also a structural component. Glial cells, supportive cells in the nervous system that were once thought to be passive bystanders, become activated and release inflammatory molecules that further sensitize pain pathways.[8] This neuroinflammation doesn't show up on standard imaging. But it's very real, and it can keep the system locked in a state of chronic pain.

Central sensitization is the mechanism behind many chronic pain conditions. This would include, but is not limited to, fibromyalgia, complex regional pain syndrome (CRPS), and some forms of chronic low back pain. It's also why two people with similar injuries can have vastly different pain experiences. If one person's nervous system becomes centrally sensitized and the other's doesn't, the first person may continue to suffer long after the tissue has healed, while the second recovers fully.

Understanding central sensitization is crucial because it shifts the focus from "What's damaged?" to "Why is my nervous system stuck in this state?" And once we understand that, we can begin to address it. However, before we explore solutions, there's another layer to this story. This one happens even before pain signals reach the brain.

The Spinal Gate: Pain's First Filter

Pain doesn't travel directly from the body to the brain. Before it reaches conscious awareness, it passes through a spinal cord checkpoint where pain signals are processed. Once they pass here, the brain determines what to do with it. The concept is called gate control theory, and it was one of the most revolutionary ideas in pain science when it was proposed in 1965 by Ronald Melzack and Patrick Wall.[9]

The basic idea is that the spinal cord contains a "gate" that can either allow pain signals to pass through to the brain or block them, depending on what else is happening in the nervous system at that moment. The gate isn't a physical structure. It's a functional process involving neurons in the dorsal horn of the spinal cord.

Here's how it works. When you injure yourself, such as stubbing your toe, pain signals (carried by small, slow nerve fibers called C fibers and $A\delta$ [A-delta] fibers) are sent from the injury site to the spinal cord. Other sensory signals, however, such as touch and pressure, travel along larger, faster fibers called $A\beta$ (A-beta) fibers. These non-painful signals can activate inhibitory neurons in the spinal cord, which effectively "close the gate" and reduce pain signals to the brain.[10]

This is why rubbing an injured area often helps alleviate the pain. The touch sensation travels faster than the pain signal and activates the gate mechanism, temporarily blocking some of the pain from reaching the brain. It's why techniques like massage, vibration, kinesiology tape, or even transcutaneous electrical nerve stimulation (TENS) can provide relief, as they all work by stimulating those larger sensory fibers and closing the gate.[11]

However, the gate isn't controlled solely by signals coming from the body. The brain can also send signals to the spinal cord, influencing whether the gate is open or closed. This is called descending modulation. And it's one of the most powerful ways the brain regulates pain.[12]

When you're calm, distracted, or feeling safe, the brain can send inhibitory signals to the spinal cord, closing the gate and reducing pain.

This is why distraction works. When you're focused on something else, your brain allocates fewer resources to processing pain, and the gate partially closes. You've probably joked before about helping someone forget about their knee pain by breaking their finger. Not quite how it works, but it's a funny illustration of the principle: introduce a bigger alarm, and the brain temporarily ignores the smaller one.

On the other hand, when you're stressed, anxious, or afraid, the brain can send signals that open the gate, amplifying pain. This is one reason why fear and catastrophizing exacerbate pain. The brain interprets the fear as evidence of threat, opens the gate, and the pain intensifies.[13] We'll explore this dynamic in much greater depth in Chapter 3, when we talk about the emotional brain.

The body's own pain-relieving chemicals also influence the spinal gate control mechanism. The brain can release endogenous opioids. These are natural painkillers, such as endorphins, that bind to receptors in the spinal cord and dampen pain transmission.[14] This is part of the reason why the placebo effect works. When you believe you've received pain relief, your brain releases these chemicals, and the pain genuinely decreases.

Gate control theory was groundbreaking because it demonstrated that pain is more than a simple input-output system. It showed that it is actively regulated at multiple levels. Pain signals don't just travel from the body to the brain in a straight line. They're filtered and modulated, shaping them along the way. And the brain isn't a passive receiver. It's actually an active participant in determining the level of pain you experience.

This sets the stage for understanding how chronic pain develops. When the gate stays open for too long, the nervous system may lose its ability to manage pain effectively. Regardless of whether it's due to repeated injury, chronic stress, or central sensitization, the system becomes stuck in a state of hypervigilance, interpreting normal sensations as dangerous and amplifying pain signals that should have been filtered out.

Now that we understand how pain signals are regulated at the spinal level, let's examine what happens when these signals reach the brain. As well as how the brain's own network of regions interprets and amplifies signals, sometimes generating pain on its own.

The Brain's Pain Network

Pain is processed through several key areas in the brain. Each contributes to a different dimension of the experience. When a pain signal reaches the brain, it first passes through the thalamus, which acts like an air traffic controller for sensory signals.[15] The thalamus doesn't generate pain itself, but it routes incoming information to the appropriate brain regions for further processing.

From there, the signal is distributed to:

The somatosensory cortex, which tells you where the pain is, how strong it feels, and what kind of sensation it carries, such as sharp, dull, burning, or aching. This is where your cortical body maps exist, the brain's internal representation of your physical body.[16] We'll explore these maps in depth in the next section. But for now, know that this region is responsible for the "sensory-discriminative" aspect of pain. It's the part that says, "This hurts, and it's coming from my left shoulder."

The limbic system, particularly structures such as the amygdala and anterior cingulate cortex, interprets the emotional meaning of the pain.[17] The limbic system doesn't just register the pain. It judges it. Maybe you're afraid of the pain, or frustrated by it. Or perhaps you even interpret it as a sign of severe damage. This system amplifies the signal. Pain becomes not just a sensation, but a source of suffering.[18] We'll explore the limbic system's role in pain more deeply in Chapter 3, where we discuss how emotion and memory shape the pain experience.

The prefrontal cortex, which handles the thinking side of pain, is involved in what you believe about it, how you focus on it, and what you expect to happen next. This is where cognitive factors, such as attention, expectation, and meaning, come into play.[19] The prefrontal cortex doesn't just react to pain; it also predicts it. When you expect pain, whether from past experience or from being told something will hurt, the prefrontal cortex primes the rest of the brain to perceive pain. Sometimes, even before the stimulus arrives. Again, we'll explore this predictive aspect more deeply in Chapter 3.

The insula, a region tucked deep within the brain, plays a crucial role in interoception, or, in other words, your sense of the internal state of your body.[20] The insula tracks things like heart rate, breathing, temperature, and gut sensations. It's also heavily involved in processing pain and integrating it with emotional and bodily awareness. When the insula becomes overactive, even normal internal sensations can feel threatening or painful.[21]

These brain regions don't operate in isolation. They constantly communicate with one another, reinforcing each other's signals. This results in them shaping how pain is felt and interpreted. The more frequently pain shows up, the more entangled these systems become.

The thalamus routes the message, the somatosensory cortex maps the location, the limbic system infuses it with emotion, and the prefrontal cortex determines the appropriate response. This is how pain isn't just a physical sensation. It's cognitive, emotional, and experiential.

But pain doesn't stop at the brain. The brain also sends signals back down to the body, influencing the intensity of pain you feel. This is where the autonomic nervous system comes into play.

The autonomic nervous system regulates all the body's automatic functions: heart rate, blood pressure, digestion, breathing, and sweating. It consists of two branches: the sympathetic nervous system, which activates during stress and prepares you for fight-or-flight, and the parasympathetic nervous system, which promotes rest, digestion, and recovery.[22]

In cases of chronic pain and trauma, the sympathetic nervous system often becomes overactive. Even though there is no immediate danger, this can leave the body in a state of constant alertness. You may experience symptoms that appear unrelated to their pain, such as a rapid heart rate, sweating, digestive issues, fatigue, and dizziness. These symptoms are not separate problems. Instead, they are all manifestations of the same dysregulated system.[23]

This is why pain conditions often come with a host of "non-pain" symptoms. It's also why interventions that calm the autonomic nervous system, such as deep breathing, meditation, or gentle movement, can reduce pain. When the nervous system shifts out of fight-or-flight mode, the brain interprets the body as safer. And then pain often decreases.[24]

For now, it's not important to memorize the names of these regions. What matters is understanding how these parts of the brain work together to create the experience of pain. Then you can understand how that experience can be reshaped. The nervous system is powerful, but it's also malleable. Pain can be learned, but it can also be unlearned. And that process begins with understanding how the brain maps the body.

Cortical Maps and Proprioception

Inside your brain, the sensory and motor cortex houses a dynamic map of your entire body. The location of your body parts, their movements, and the sensations they experience are all represented in this map. This is what allows you to touch your nose with your eyes closed or feel your foot on the gas pedal without needing to look.

That sense is called proprioception, which is your awareness of your body's position in space.[25] The most common visual representation of the brain's body map is the homunculus. This is a strange-looking human figure with disproportionately large hands, lips, and eyes. It illustrates how much brain space is allocated to different body parts based on the amount of sensory input they provide. Areas with more nerve endings and constant sensory feedback, such as the hands and mouth, occupy a significantly larger portion of the brain's map.

If you've never seen it, look it up. It's odd, even comical at first glance, but it gives you a powerful visual of how your brain prioritizes sensation.

While proprioception is a sensory ability, it feeds into the sensory and motor cortex, which then updates your brain's body map. This map is flexible and constantly adapting. However, that flexibility comes at a cost, as it can become altered if the input remains unchanged for too long.

Now imagine what happens when one area starts sending only pain signals. If a joint stops moving smoothly, a muscle stops being used, starts overcompensating, or any other catastrophic signal floods the brain from a particular region, the map for that area can become blurred, enlarged, or amplified. The brain starts over-monitoring that region, treating normal sensations as a threat. Once this "threat" is perceived, the brain gives that area heightened attention. The map becomes maladapted, amplifying signals from that part of the body and reinforcing the pain loop. This is how chronic pain begins to override accurate perception.

But the brain doesn't just map your body's position in space. It also monitors internal activity, including your heart rate, breathing, gut sensations, and muscle tension. In other words, it's what you feel inside your body, such as being tired, hungry, emotional, and in pain. This is what we mentioned earlier, called interoception, and it's just as critical to how you experience pain.[26] Again, interoception is processed primarily in the insula, which is also heavily involved in pain perception. When interoceptive signals are misread, such as an elevated heart rate being interpreted as danger rather than exertion, the brain can amplify pain as a protective response.[27]

Chronic pain patients often have altered interoception. They're more sensitive to internal sensations and more likely to interpret them as threatening.[28] This is why chronic pain can come with a pervasive sense of "something is wrong," despite medical tests showing nothing abnormal. The brain's internal monitoring system becomes hypersensitive. And that hypersensitivity feeds into the pain experience.

This is how what begins as a localized issue can grow to feel overwhelming, even when the damage is no longer evident. This alteration doesn't just affect our perception of pain but also how it manifests in the body, especially through trigger points and referred pain patterns.

Trigger Points and Referred Pain

Trigger points are among the clearest real-world examples of how altered cortical maps can manifest in the body. These hyperirritable spots in muscle tissue don't just cause local pain. They often refer pain to entirely different areas. Press on a trigger point in your neck, and you might feel pain radiate down your shoulder or even into your head.

Some classic examples are trigger points in the glutes that refer pain down the leg. Or you may have a trigger point in the upper shoulder that sends pain into the head and behind the eye. These are a couple of examples among myriad ways this can play out.

These patterns are common enough to be documented in medical charts. Clinically, trigger points have been mapped with remarkable consistency across most of the population; approximately 75% to 80% of people tend to exhibit similar referral patterns.[29] But these aren't rules carved in stone. There are always exceptions. Some people feel referred pain in different areas, or not at all. That variation is important, and it supports the idea that your brain's interpretation of the pain signal matters just as much as the location where the signal originates.

Initially, it was believed that referred pain followed strict nerve pathways. And it is often still taught in this manner in many manual therapy courses. But we now understand that the brain's interpretation of nociceptive input (pain-related signals) plays a significant role.[30] This is leading to the growing recognition that trigger points may be more neuroplastic than strictly mechanical.

Now, this doesn't mean trigger points are "all in your head" or that the local tissue dysfunction isn't real. Trigger points have historically been explained as localized muscle dysfunction. Tight bands of muscle fibers can cause ischemia (a lack of oxygen in tissue). This leads to the accumulation of metabolic waste, which is typically the cause of trigger points. But referred pain patterns can vary between individuals. Trigger points can even persist after tissue normalization. This suggests a central component. Research on central sensitization in musculoskeletal pain supports this view, showing that the nervous system's amplification of signals can maintain trigger points even after peripheral dysfunction resolves.[31]

In other words, the pain that trigger points produce isn't always tied to direct anatomical structures. It often reflects how the brain interprets and organizes sensory input, sometimes even altering it.

This aligns with my current view, which is that referred pain from trigger points is frequently shaped not by precise nerve pathways, but by alterations in the brain's internal body map. As the brain gives more attention to a region in distress, that area can become amplified and blurred in the cortical map. This means even normal or mild sensations may be interpreted as painful. This isn't an exaggeration. It's a great example of how the brain prioritizes what it perceives as a threat. And by doing so, it reinforces those pathways until they dominate perception.

Here's how this works in practice. The part of the brain that maps your shoulder sits right next to the part that maps your upper arm, which sits next to the region for your forearm, and then your hand. These regions are neighbors on the cortical map. When a trigger point in your shoulder becomes active, and the brain amplifies that region, the signal doesn't stay neatly contained. It smears across the map, influencing neighboring areas. The brain's representation of your shoulder "bleeds" into the map for your arm.[32] This is why a knot in your shoulder can produce pain that travels down your entire arm, even when the peripheral tissues in your arm are perfectly fine. There may be a peripheral component, sure. The nerve pathways are sending signals. But the brain's map has reorganized. This is the reason you feel pain in the arm rather than just tension in the shoulder. The boundary's blurred, and what started as a localized problem has become a regional one. Not because the tissue damage spreads, but because the brain's interpretation of that region expands over time. This can lead to central sensitization, in which the nervous system becomes more responsive to input.[33] We'll explore how this process manifests in conditions like fibromyalgia and Ehlers-Danlos Syndrome in later chapters.

Pulling It Together

Now, we can see maladaptive neuroplasticity at work across every system we've explored.

Central sensitization is the nervous system learning to amplify signals. It's turning the volume up so high that even normal sensations register as pain. The spinal gate remaining open when it should be closed is an example of learned spinal cord hypersensitivity. Repeated pain signals have trained the system to let everything through. Altered cortical maps are the brain reorganizing itself around threat signals or enlarging the representation of painful areas, leading regular input to be misread as danger. Trigger points that refer pain in unexpected patterns are remapping pathways in action, with the brain rewriting the rules about where pain should be felt.

These aren't separate problems. They're expressions aren't the same underlying process. The nervous system has become exceptionally good at producing pain because it's practiced doing so repeatedly.

For example, after an amputation, the brain doesn't simply "turn off" the region that used to represent the "missing limb". Instead, surrounding brain areas begin to invade that unused cortical territory.[34] Adjacent regions, like the face or the remaining arm, start to take over the space that once belonged to the missing hand or foot. This cortical reorganization is directly linked to the intensity of phantom pain. Research shows that the more extensive this invasion, the more severe the pain tends to be.[35]

What's striking is that this process can be reversed. Mirror therapy, which uses visual feedback to convince the brain that the limb is still present and moving without pain, has been shown to reduce phantom limb pain by helping the brain rewire itself.[36] The brain's map isn't fixed. It changes based on input, use, and experience. And once it changes, those changes can persist long after the original trigger is gone.

The same principle applies to other forms of chronic pain. Studies of people with chronic low back pain have found that the region of the somatosensory cortex representing the back becomes "smeared" or less distinct, as if the brain has lost its precise map of that area.[37] This blurring correlates with pain intensity and can persist even when the tissue itself has healed. The map has been redrawn, and the brain continues to interpret signals from that region as threatening or painful.

Traditionally, neuroplasticity refers to the brain and spinal cord's ability to reorganize themselves, a property of the central nervous system. However, in this book, we use the term more broadly. The changes don't stop at the spinal cord. Peripheral nerves, which run from your spinal cord to your skin, muscles, and organs, can also rewire.[38] After an injury, nerve endings can become more excitable, firing more easily and more often.[39] In some cases, damaged nerves can even grow new branches (a process called sprouting), creating abnormal connections that send chaotic signals back to the spinal cord and brain.[40]

Imagine you're tuning a radio. When you're one frequency from the station you want, you may still catch fragments of that broadcast. But it's riddled with static and overlapping noise from adjacent channels. The signal is present, but it's unclear and confusing. That's what happens when nerves sprout and create new, unintended pathways. The information is real, but the way it's processed creates chaos.

These peripheral changes don't exist in isolation. They talk back to the brain, which then reinforces them, creating a feedback loop that can lead to chronic pain.[41] So when we talk about neuroplasticity in this book, we mean the entire nervous system's ability to adapt, for better or worse. It's all one conversation.

Pain becomes a habit. The nervous system becomes efficient at producing it. Even when the tissue improves, the signal may persist. The story of chronic pain isn't about being broken or weak. It's about how powerful the brain is at learning. And if pain can be learned, it can also be unlearned. That's what the rest of this book will explore: how pain patterns are reinforced, how they persist, and how they can begin to change.

In the next chapter, we'll explore how these reinforced patterns form self-sustaining feedback loops, making them even more challenging to break. We'll explore the pain loop, examining how pain not only persists but also feeds on itself.

Reflection Prompt

Take a moment to think about a time when your pain didn't make any sense. Perhaps it appeared in an unusual place, or lingered long after the injury had healed. How did that experience affect the way you trusted your body? Did it make you doubt yourself? Feel dismissed by others? Keep this in mind as we move forward. These experiences are part of the story we're working to reframe.

Endnotes

[1] Apkarian, A. V., Baliki, M. N., & Geha, P. Y. (2009). Towards a theory of chronic pain. Progress in Neurobiology, 87(2):81-97.

[2] Flor, H., Elbert, T., Knecht, S., et al. (1995). *Phantom-limb pain as a perceptual correlate of cortical reorganization following arm amputation.* Nature, 375, 482–484.

[3] Woolf, C. J. (2011). Central sensitization: Implications for the diagnosis and treatment of pain. *Pain*, 152(3), S2–S15.

[4] Latremoliere, A., & Woolf, C. J. (2009). Central sensitization: A generator of pain hypersensitivity by central neural plasticity. *Journal of Pain*, 10(9), 895–926.

[5] Herrero, J. F., Laird, J. M., & López-García, J. A. (2000). Wind-up of spinal cord neurones and pain sensation: Much ado about something? *Progress in Neurobiology*, 61(2), 169–203.

[6] Sandkühler, J. (2009). Models and mechanisms of hyperalgesia and allodynia. *Physiological Reviews*, 89(2), 707–758.

[7] Woolf, C. J., & Salter, M. W. (2000). Neuronal plasticity: Increasing the gain in pain. *Science*, 288(5472), 1765–1769.

[8] Ji, R. R., Berta, T., & Nedergaard, M. (2013). Glia and pain: Is chronic pain a gliopathy? *Pain*, 154(Suppl 1), S10–S28.

[9] Melzack, R., & Wall, P. D. (1965). Pain mechanisms: A new theory. *Science*, 150(3699), 971–979.

[10] Mendell, L. M. (2014). Constructing and deconstructing the gate theory of pain. *Pain*, 155(2), 210–216.

[11] Johnson, M. I., Paley, C. A., Howe, T. E., & Sluka, K. A. (2015). Transcutaneous electrical nerve stimulation for acute pain. *Cochrane Database of Systematic Reviews*, 6, CD006142.

[12] Ossipov, M. H., Dussor, G. O., & Porreca, F. (2010). Central modulation of pain. *Journal of Clinical Investigation*, 120(11), 3779–3787.

[13] Leeuw, M., Goossens, M. E., Linton, S. J., Crombez, G., Boersma, K., & Vlaeyen, J. W. (2007). The fear-avoidance model of musculoskeletal pain: Current state of scientific evidence. *Journal of Behavioral Medicine*, 30(1), 77–94.

[14] Fields, H. L. (2004). State-dependent opioid control of pain. *Nature Reviews Neuroscience*, 5(7), 565–575.

[15] Apkarian, A. V., Bushnell, M. C., Treede, R. D., & Zubieta, J. K. (2005). Human brain mechanisms of pain perception and regulation in health and disease. *European Journal of Pain*, 9(4), 463–484.

[16] Penfield, W., & Boldrey, E. (1937). Somatic motor and sensory representation in the cerebral cortex of man as

studied by electrical stimulation. *Brain*, 60(4), 389–443.

[17] Rainville, P., Duncan, G. H., Price, D. D., Carrier, B., & Bushnell, M. C. (1997). Pain affect encoded in human anterior cingulate but not somatosensory cortex. *Science*, 277(5328), 968–971.

[18] Bushnell, M. C., Ceko, M., & Low, L. A. (2013). Cognitive and emotional control of pain and its disruption in chronic pain. *Nature Reviews Neuroscience*, 14(7), 502–511.

[19] Tracey, I., & Mantyh, P. W. (2007). The cerebral signature for pain perception and its modulation. *Neuron*, 55(3), 377–391.

[20] Craig, A. D. (2003). Interoception: The sense of the physiological condition of the body. *Current Opinion in Neurobiology*, 13(4), 500–505.

[21] Paulus, M. P., & Stein, M. B. (2010). Interoception in anxiety and depression. *Brain Structure and Function*, 214(5-6), 451–463.

[22] Porges, S. W. (2011). *The Polyvagal Theory: Neurophysiological Foundations of Emotions, Attachment, Communication, and Self-regulation*. W. W. Norton & Company.

[23] Nijs, J., Leysen, L., Vanlauwe, J., Logghe, T., Ickmans, K., Polli, A., Malfliet, A., Coppieters, I., & Huysmans, E. (2019). Treatment of central sensitization in patients with chronic pain: Time for change? *Expert Opinion on Pharmacotherapy*, 20(16), 1961–1970.

[24] Khoury, B., Sharma, M., Rush, S. E., & Fournier, C. (2015). Mindfulness-based stress reduction for healthy individuals: A meta-analysis. *Journal of Psychosomatic Research*, 78(6), 519–528.

[25] Proske, U., & Gandevia, S. C. (2012). The proprioceptive senses: Their roles in signaling body shape, body position and movement, and muscle force. *Physiological Reviews*, 92(4), 1651–1697.

[26] Craig, A. D. (2002). How do you feel? Interoception: The sense of the physiological condition of the body. *Nature Reviews Neuroscience*, 3(8), 655–666.

[27] Critchley, H. D., Wiens, S., Rotshtein, P., Öhman, A., & Dolan, R. J. (2004). Neural systems supporting interoceptive awareness. *Nature Neuroscience*, 7(2), 189–195.

[28] Di Lernia, D., Serino, S., & Riva, G. (2016). Pain in the body. Altered interoception in chronic pain conditions: A systematic review. *Neuroscience & Biobehavioral Reviews*, 71, 328–341.

[29] Simons, D. G., Travell, J. G., & Simons, L. S. (1999). *Travell & Simons' Myofascial Pain and Dysfunction: The Trigger Point Manual* (2nd ed.). Williams & Wilkins.

[30] Giamberardino, M. A., Affaitati, G., Fabrizio, A., & Costantini, R. (2011). Myofascial pain syndromes and their evaluation. *Best Practice & Research Clinical Rheumatology*, 25(2), 185–198.

[31] Nijs, J., Van Houdenhove, B., & Oostendorp, R. A. (2010). Recognition of central sensitization in patients with musculoskeletal pain: Application of pain neurophysiology in manual therapy practice. *Manual Therapy*, 15(2), 135–141.

[32] Flor, H., Braun, C., Elbert, T., & Birbaumer, N. (1997). Extensive reorganization of primary somatosensory cortex in chronic back pain patients. *Neuroscience Letters*, 224(1), 5–8.

[33] Yunus, M. B. (2007). Role of central sensitization in symptoms of fibromyalgia. *The American Journal of Medicine*, 120(Suppl 1), S3–S13.

[34] Flor, H., Elbert, T., Knecht, S., Wienbruch, C., Pantev, C., Birbaumer, N., Larbig, W., & Taub, E. (1995). Phantom-limb pain as a perceptual correlate of cortical reorganization following arm amputation. *Nature*, 375(6531), 482–484.

[35] Birbaumer, N., Lutzenberger, W., Montoya, P., Larbig, W., Unertl, K., Töpfner, S., Grodd, W., Taub, E., & Flor, H. (1997). Effects of regional anesthesia on phantom limb pain are mirrored in changes in cortical reorganization. *Journal of Neuroscience*, 17(14), 5503–5508.

[36] Ramachandran, V. S., & Altschuler, E. L. (2009). The use of visual feedback, in particular mirror visual feedback, in restoring brain function. *Brain*, 132(7), 1693–1710.

[37] Flor, H., Braun, C., Elbert, T., & Birbaumer, N. (1997). Extensive reorganization of primary somatosensory cortex in chronic back pain patients. *Neuroscience Letters*, 224(1), 5–8.

[38] Woolf, C. J., & Ma, Q. (2007). Nociceptors—noxious stimulus detectors. *Neuron*, 55(3), 353–364.

[39] Basbaum, A. I., Bautista, D. M., Scherrer, G., & Julius, D. (2009). Cellular and molecular mechanisms of pain. *Cell*, 139(2), 267–284.

[40] Doubell, T. P., Mannion, R. J., & Woolf, C. J. (1999). The dorsal horn: State-dependent sensory processing, plasticity, and the generation of pain. In *Textbook of Pain* (4th ed., pp. 165–181). Churchill Livingstone.

[41] Costigan, M., Scholz, J., & Woolf, C. J. (2009). Neuropathic pain: A maladaptive response of the nervous system to damage. *Annual Review of Neuroscience*, 32, 1–32.

Chapter 2

Why Pain Persists

Pain doesn't just happen. It follows patterns. And once those patterns are set, they become the brain's default response. This is one of the most essential truths in chronic pain. It's not just about what happened to your body. It's about what your brain learned from it and what it continues to expect. In Chapter One, we explored how the brain interprets pain and how it can feel confusing or disconnected from injury. Here, we build on that foundation to explain why those signals persist.

The nervous system is efficient. It reinforces what it uses most. Each time a pain signal travels through your system, the pathway becomes a little stronger. Over time, pain can become the path of least resistance, the route your brain takes automatically.[1] Even after the original injury has healed, the signal may continue firing because the system has become so proficient at sending it. Once these patterns are established, they often feed into a self-reinforcing cycle. We'll call it the pain loop.

This is maladaptive neuroplasticity in action: the same ability that allows us to learn new skills and habits can also cement pain pathways.[2] Just like practicing an instrument strengthens muscle memory, repeated pain reinforces the brain's pain memory. Eventually, it takes less and less stimulus to trigger the response. Sometimes, the brain can even interpret neutral signals, or no signal at all, as a form of pain.

Think of it like this. If you decide to go walking through the woods, the first time you cut through the trees, it's rough. The ground is uneven, and branches are in your way. But the more often you take that route, the clearer it becomes. The grass flattens, the dirt hardens, the trail becomes obvious. Eventually, it's the easiest way through the forest.

That's what happens in your nervous system. Pain becomes the worn path. Not necessarily the right path, but the one that's easiest to follow.

This doesn't mean peripheral factors don't matter. Inflammation, tissue damage, and structural issues are real. But even after those heal, the nervous system can keep signaling pain. This is because the pathway has become so well-established. These physical factors initially carve the trail, or at least shape its formation. But neuroplasticity is what keeps it clear and easy to follow long after the original threat has passed.

Pain patterns can start in many ways. For instance, an injury can heal physically but leave behind an established signal. Postural imbalances or poor movement habits can repeatedly stress the same tissues, setting off the pattern. Another example is overuse syndromes that constantly irritate muscles or joints, or even muscle weakness that forces the body to compensate inefficiently. Even lifestyle factors like poor sleep, high stress, or chronic inflammation can lower the threshold for pain perception.[3]

Why some people transition from acute to chronic pain while others recover fully isn't entirely understood. Research suggests there is a combination of factors, such as genetics, prior pain experiences, stress levels, sleep quality, psychological resilience, and even early life trauma. Any of these can all influence whether pain pathways become deeply entrenched or fade as tissues heal.[4] Some nervous systems seem more prone to sensitization than others, though we don't yet know all the reasons why. This isn't about weakness or failure. It's about how your particular system responds to threat, and that response is shaped by biology, history, and circumstance.

In each of these cases, the initial signal is real. But the longer it fires, the more entrenched it becomes. Over time, the body adapts, but not always in helpful ways. Compensatory movement patterns reinforce the problem, feeding more input into the same pain pathways. Even when tissues recover, the signal may continue because the brain has learned to expect it. Once these signals take hold, they don't just remain. They build momentum.

You see this play out everywhere in daily life. Someone who sits for eight hours a day at a desk may notice their back and neck tightening into a spasm by late afternoon. Poor sleep after a stressful day can leave you waking stiff, literally as though your body rehearsed tension all night long. A weekend warrior may strain a calf playing basketball. Even though the muscle heals in a few weeks, he may still limp months later. Not because the tissue is injured, but because the nervous system has reinforced the protective pathway. These lived experiences help explain why so many people feel pain even when nothing "new" is happening.

The Pain-Spasm Cycle

One of the clearest examples of this reinforcement loop is the pain-spasm cycle. Here's how the worn path plays out in your muscles.

Pain or perceived threat. The nervous system responds by guarding. Muscles tighten to protect the area.

Guarding and spasm. Tight muscles restrict blood flow and oxygen. Metabolites (waste products from muscle activity) build up, tissues stiffen, and local nerves become more sensitive.[5]

Sensitized input. Those irritated tissues send louder signals. The brain turns up its internal "gain," interpreting more activity as a threat. This "gain" refers to how sensitized the nervous system becomes. In chronic pain, areas like the anterior cingulate cortex and insula, which process threat and emotional meaning, become hyperactive.[6] The threshold for what counts as "dangerous" drops. Signals that would typically be filtered out as background noise now get flagged as threats, amplifying the pain experience.

More pain. Your body doubles down on guarding, and the cycle repeats.

The longer this runs, the more efficient the pathway becomes. The nervous system is doing what it's designed to do: learn from repetition.[7] A poor night's sleep, or even a long drive, minor stressors over time can trip the same alarm.

And because guarding often comes with fear, the cycle tightens further. "If I move wrong, it'll hurt more." That thought alone can immobilize you. Your body stays locked with you. The pathway deepens.

Stress hormones, such as cortisol and adrenaline, can lower pain thresholds and keep the nervous system in a heightened state of alert when they are chronically elevated.[8] This biochemical shift makes it easier for the pain-spasm cycle to trip, even with minor triggers. The body's stress response has evolved to protect us from immediate danger. But this becomes a liability when it fails to shut off entirely. We'll explore this connection between stress and pain in much greater depth in the next chapter.

Trigger Points and Why Pain Travels

This is also the environment where latent trigger points tend to become active. We introduced trigger points in Chapter One as hyper-irritable spots that refer pain unpredictably. Now let's see how they fit into the pain loop. While the exact mechanisms are still debated in research, clinically, we observe a pattern. Latent points don't constantly hurt on their own.[9] You mainly feel them when pressed, or as stiffness and weakness. In practice, I can push on a latent point and create a referral pattern even though the client wasn't feeling it before. This suggests that these points exist and can be activated, even if the complete picture of how and why isn't universally agreed upon in the literature.

When guarding persists, circulation decreases, and metabolites accumulate. High stress or movement avoidance can trigger those latent points to become active. Once active, they send a cascade of pain signals to the brain, generating spontaneous pain and broader referral patterns. A small knot in one region spreads discomfort across a much larger area.

Why does the pain seem to travel? Part of it is peripheral. The irritated muscle and surrounding tissues are genuinely more sensitive. Part of it is central. The brain's map for that region becomes more responsive and starts assigning a broader area to the same perceived threat.[10]

This ties back to Chapter One's explanation of cortical maps. Traditionally, referred pain from trigger points has been explained through peripheral nerve pathways. However, there is growing evidence that cortical mapping plays a more significant role. The brain misinterprets and amplifies signals, spreading them across regions that are linked in its sensory map.[11] This is why a small source of irritation can feel like pain spreading far beyond its origin.

Again, this doesn't mean the pain is imagined. It means the brain has become more efficient at assigning threat to a larger area. Over time, this mechanism can cause pain to feel exaggerated and more dominant than its source. Common everyday examples include a shoulder knot triggering headaches or back tension radiating into the hips.

These patterns follow conventional anatomical expectations. But what about when they don't?

My theory is that trigger points themselves are neuroplastic in nature. When the brain's body map becomes altered through chronic pain or trauma, the referral patterns can break from conventional anatomical expectations entirely. This is why, in conditions like fibromyalgia, I might push on someone's hip, and they'll feel pain in their shoulder. This would be a referral pattern that doesn't follow traditional nerve pathways or dermatomes. The brain has rewritten the map, and the signal gets routed through pathways that wouldn't make sense under conventional thinking. We'll explore this idea in much greater depth when we discuss fibromyalgia and other complex pain conditions in later chapters. But for now, understand that the plasticity we're describing doesn't just amplify pain. It can fundamentally rewire where and how you feel it.

The good news is that as the loop is de-escalated and healthier movement, circulation, and new input return, those active points often quiet back down. Sometimes reverting to a latent state, or even resolving altogether. We'll return to this idea of cortical involvement in later chapters, especially when we dig into fibromyalgia and other complex pain conditions.

Understanding Hurt vs. Harm

This cycle is learned and reinforced through repetition rather than being locked in by permanent damage. This is encouraging because it can also be interrupted. That's where treatment comes in. But here's the thing you have to understand. Breaking a well-worn path isn't about one big intervention. It's about giving the nervous system consistent, repeated signals that provide an alternative route.

This is where understanding the difference between "hurt" and "harm" becomes crucial. Pain is a warning signal. But in chronic conditions, it's often a false alarm.[12] The system has become so sensitive that it fires even when there's no ongoing tissue damage. Something can cause intense pain without causing harm. That distinction is what allows movement and activity to be safe, even when they're uncomfortable.

For the record, I am not suggesting you tough it out or force yourself to move through it. I get it. That's what you have been hearing from everyone else around you, with little to no understanding of your situation. However, it is the conceptual foundation that allows you to begin to trust your body again, to move despite pain, and to gradually teach your nervous system that the threat it's perceiving isn't real.

Let me give you some real-world examples of what this looks like. Someone with chronic back pain might feel a sharp twinge when bending to pick up a pencil. That twinge isn't telling them their spine is breaking. It's their nervous system overreacting to movement that it's learned to associate with threat. The tissue can handle the load just fine. The alarm system is malfunctioning.

Or consider someone who's been avoiding stairs for months because their knee doesn't feel right. The cartilage might be perfectly intact, and the muscles might be strong enough. But the brain has flagged that movement as dangerous, so it amplifies those sensations into pain. The hurt is real, even if the harm isn't there.

This distinction matters. It shifts the approach from "avoid everything that hurts" to "gradually retrain the system to recognize safe movement." You're not denying the pain; you're teaching your nervous system that the alarm can be turned down. You're teaching it that the threat it's warning you about doesn't actually exist.

This concept bridges the understanding of why pain persists and the ability to interrupt it. It's also why many people get stuck. They interpret all pain as a sign of damage, so they stop moving and stop engaging. This gives the nervous system exactly the kind of input that reinforces the cycle. Stillness confirms the threat. Movement, done gradually and mindfully, challenges it.

Movement as Signal

Here's something that often gets missed in pain management. Movement isn't just physical rehabilitation. It's communication with your nervous system. Every time you move, you're sending signals to your brain about what's safe and what's not. And your brain is listening.

When you avoid movement because of pain, you're sending a clear message: "This area is dangerous. Stay on high alert." The nervous system responds by maintaining or even increasing its protective response. Muscles stay tight. The brain's body map for that region remains amplified. The pain pathway stays well-worn.

But when you move, carefully, gradually, and within safe limits, you're sending a different signal: "This area is safe. You can relax the guard." There's a critical difference here. Moving through discomfort is not the same as pushing through sharp, stabbing pain. Nor is forcing your body past danger signals. Discomfort is the feeling of challenge, the sensation of testing an edge. Pain that feels like a warning, like something is going wrong, is different. That's your nervous system telling you to back off. What we're talking about here is the kind of movement that feels hard or uncomfortable but doesn't set off alarm bells. Over time, with consistent input at that manageable edge, the nervous system begins to believe it's safe. The alarm system recalibrates. The pain pathway weakens.

This is why graded exposure works. Graded exposure is the practice of slowly, systematically reintroducing movements or activities that have become associated with pain. But you have to start small. It could be as simple as bending forward a few degrees if that movement has been avoided. Or walking for five minutes if walking has felt impossible. You're not pushing through pain recklessly. You're testing the edges of what feels tolerable and gradually expanding them.

The goal isn't to prove you're tough. The goal is to give your nervous system new information. To show it, through repeated safe experiences, that the threat it's perceiving isn't real. Each time you move without catastrophe, the brain updates its prediction. The association between movement and danger begins to loosen.[13]

This is also why prolonged rest often backfires. Rest can be helpful in the acute phase of an injury, when tissues genuinely need time to heal. But when rest extends beyond that healing window, it becomes a problem. The brain never gets new information to challenge the old threat pattern. The body map for the rested area becomes less defined. Muscles start to weaken. The nervous system becomes hypersensitive and out of practice. And when you finally do try to move again, the nervous system overreacts. The pain flares, and the cycle deepens.

Think of it this way. If you stop using a language, you forget how to speak it fluently. If you stop moving a part of your body, your brain forgets how to move it without alarm. Movement keeps the map clear and the pathways active. Most of all, it keeps the system calibrated. It's not just about strength or flexibility. It's about maintaining the brain's confidence in the body.

This doesn't mean you should force yourself into movements that feel genuinely dangerous or that cause sharp, escalating pain. That's not the kind of signal we're talking about. What we're describing is the gradual reintroduction of movement within a tolerable range, with the understanding that discomfort doesn't always mean damage. You're teaching the system through experience, not willpower.

We'll explore specific strategies for graded movement and pacing in the third section of this book, where we discuss interventions in detail. For now, the key takeaway is this. Movement isn't just a treatment. It's a language. And the more clearly you can speak it, the more your nervous system will listen.

Breaking the Cycle

So, how do you actually interrupt the pain loop? The short answer is: consistently, gradually, and from multiple angles. The nervous system doesn't respond well to one-off interventions. It responds to repetition. And it will respond to variety as well as new patterns that compete with the old ones.

This is why many treatments can provide relief, though often temporarily at first. Muscle relaxers work by reducing spasm, so the cycle doesn't tighten further. Manual therapy calms hyperactive muscles and restores circulation, interrupting the buildup of metabolites that perpetuate pain.[14] Corrective exercise introduces new and healthier movement input, challenging the pain network to adopt different pathways. Even kinesiology taping or mindful movement practices can alter the brain's feedback loop long enough to dampen it.

Each of these tools is, in its own way, an attempt to break the pain-spasm cycle and interrupt the signal that keeps it looping. They may look different on the surface, but they share a common goal: interrupt the loop. Without repetition and reinforcement, however, the nervous system tends to revert to its default. The easier route is already known.

Overwriting a signal that's been reinforced for months or years isn't about one big breakthrough. It's about consistent input over time. You need to feed the system new information repeatedly until the older pain response becomes less dominant. After a while, a new response pattern begins to take hold.[15] You need stronger, clearer signals, repeated often enough, to carve a new path through the forest and make it the easier route for your brain and body to follow.

For some, meaningful change can occur in as little as a few weeks. For others, it may take months or even longer, especially for those with years of reinforced patterns. The timeline may vary, but the principle remains the same. Repeated input, over time, can reshape these pathways.

But recovery is rarely, if ever, linear. You'll have good days and bad days. There may be days when the pain seems to vanish. Then all of a sudden, there are days when it roars back as if nothing has changed. This isn't failure, it's part of the retraining process. The nervous system is testing the new pattern while comparing it to the old one. Then it has to decide which one to trust.

Setbacks don't erase progress. They're part of the landscape you're navigating.

What matters is the overall trend. Are the flare-ups getting less frequent? Less intense? Shorter in duration? Are you able to do more than you could a month ago, even if it's just a little? That's progress. That's the pathway shifting.

This is also why consistency matters more than intensity. A small amount of the right input, repeated daily, will outperform a heroic effort once a week. The brain learns through repetition, not through single dramatic events. Ten minutes of mindful movement every day will rewire the system more effectively than an hour-long session once in a while. This is because the brain needs frequent reminders that the new pattern is the one to follow.

And this is where patience becomes essential. You're not just treating pain. You're retraining a system that has been practicing the wrong response for a long time. That takes time and trust. And it takes the willingness to keep going, even when progress feels slow.

Common Mistakes That Keep People Stuck

Even with the best intentions, people often fall into patterns that reinforce the very cycle they're trying to break. These mistakes aren't about laziness or weakness. They're about misunderstanding how the nervous system works. And once you see them clearly, they're easier to avoid.

Relying only on passive treatments. Massage feels good. Chiropractic adjustments can provide relief. Medications can take the edge off. But if these are the only tools you're using, you're missing the bigger picture. Passive treatments can temporarily interrupt the cycle, but they don't retrain the system. They don't give your brain new information. Without active participation, without movement and engagement, the old pattern will reassert itself. You need both: passive interventions to calm the system, and active strategies to rewire it.

Resting too much. Rest is essential after an acute injury. But prolonged rest, especially when driven by fear of pain, can teach the nervous system that movement is dangerous. The more you avoid movement, the more sensitive the system becomes. When you finally do move again, the alarm bells ring louder. You'll feel worse, and then the temptation to rest will grow stronger. It's a vicious cycle. The solution isn't to push through recklessly. It's to move gradually, consistently, and within tolerable limits. To show your nervous system, through repeated safe experiences, that movement is not the enemy.

Pushing through pain recklessly. On the flip side, there's the "no pain, no gain" mentality. The belief that if you just tough it out, the pain will eventually go away. But then you push too hard and too fast. Doing so, you're not retraining the system; you're reinforcing the threat signal. The nervous system interprets that sharp escalation of pain as confirmation that it was right to be on high alert. The cycle tightens. The pathway deepens. The key is finding the edge, the place where you're challenging the system without overwhelming it. That's where retraining happens.

Expecting linear progress. Healing isn't a straight line. You'll have setbacks. You'll have days when the pain feels as bad as it ever did, even though you've been doing everything right. This doesn't mean the work isn't working, but that the nervous system is still learning. It's still comparing the new pattern to the old one. Setbacks are part of the process. What matters is the overall trend over weeks and months, not the day-to-day fluctuations.

Ignoring the role of stress and emotion. Pain doesn't exist in a vacuum. It's influenced by sleep, stress, emotional state, and nervous system regulation. If you're treating the pain but ignoring the stress that keeps your system on high alert, you're fighting an uphill battle. We'll explore this in much more depth in the next chapter. But for now, understand that calming the nervous system, not just treating the tissues, is essential.

These mistakes are understandable. They're what most people do, because they're what most people have been taught. But once you see them for what they are, roadblocks rather than solutions, you can start to move around them. And that's when progress becomes possible.

Pulling It Together

The capacity for change exists in the very system that created the problem in the first place. That doesn't mean the process is easy, or that your pain can be erased with a quick fix. It means there's a path forward. By understanding why pain persists, you can stop blaming yourself. You can stop chasing dead ends and start to see why consistency, patience, and the right tools matter. And you can begin to approach your pain not as a mystery, but as a pattern. One that can be interrupted, redirected, and eventually reshaped.

In the next chapter, we'll look more closely at how the emotional brain (the limbic system and the way you think about pain) can amplify these patterns. Stress and emotional reactivity can exacerbate the pain. And this can make it more difficult to escape. That sets the stage for understanding why patience, perspective, and consistency matter. And, why blame yourself only fuels the cycle further.

For now, hold on to this. Persistent pain is not meaningless or imaginary. It is a learned signal. And what is learned can, over time and with the right input, be unlearned.

Endnotes

[1] Latremoliere, A., & Woolf, C. J. (2009). *Central sensitization: A generator of pain hypersensitivity by central neural plasticity.* Journal of Pain, 10(9), 895–926.

[2] Moseley, G. L., & Flor, H. (2012). Targeting cortical representations in the treatment of chronic pain: A review. *Neurorehabilitation and Neural Repair*, 26(6), 646-652.

[3] Nijs, J., et al. (2015). Sleep disturbances and severe stress as glial activators: Implications for chronic pain. *Expert Review of Neurotherapeutics*, 15(5), 385-392.

[4] Diatchenko, L., et al. (2013). The phenotypic and genetic signatures of common musculoskeletal pain conditions. *Nature Reviews Rheumatology*, 9(6), 340-350.

[5] Shah, J. P., et al. (2015). Myofascial trigger points then and now: A historical and scientific perspective. *PM&R*, 7(7), 746-761.

[6] Baliki, M. N., et al. (2012). Corticostriatal functional connectivity predicts transition to chronic back pain. *Nature Neuroscience*, 15(8), 1117-1119.

[7] Woolf, C. J. (2011). Central sensitization: Implications for the diagnosis and treatment of pain. *Pain*, 152(3 Suppl), S2-S15.

[8] McEwen, B. S. (2007). Physiology and neurobiology of stress and adaptation: Central role of the brain. *Physiological Reviews*, 87(3), 873-904.

[9] Simons, D. G., Travell, J. G., & Simons, L. S. (1999). *Travell & Simons' Myofascial Pain and Dysfunction: The Trigger Point Manual* (2nd ed.). Lippincott Williams & Wilkins.

[10] Flor, H., Braun, C., Elbert, T., & Birbaumer, N. (1997). Extensive reorganization of primary somatosensory cortex in chronic back pain patients. Neuroscience Letters, 224(1), 5–8.

[11] Moseley, G. L. (2003). A pain neuromatrix approach to patients with chronic pain. *Manual Therapy*, 8(3), 130-140.

[12] Butler, D. S., & Moseley, G. L. (2013). *Explain Pain* (2nd ed.). Noigroup Publications.

[13] Louw, A., et al. (2016). The efficacy of pain neuroscience education on musculoskeletal pain: A systematic review of the literature. *Physiotherapy Theory and Practice*, 32(5), 332-355.

[14] Hou, C. R., et al. (2002). Immediate effects of various physical therapeutic modalities on cervical myofascial pain and trigger-point sensitivity. *Archives of Physical Medicine and Rehabilitation*, 83(10), 1406-1414.

[15] Doidge, N. (2007). *The Brain That Changes Itself: Stories of Personal Triumph from the Frontiers of Brain Science*. Penguin Books.

Chapter 3

The Emotional Brain

You're stuck in traffic. Your shoulders creep toward your ears. By the time you park, that familiar ache in your neck has already started. Nothing has touched you, much less injured you. But your body knew the stress was coming. And it responded as if the threats were real.

By now, we've seen how pain signals can form loops, reinforcing them over time. Chapter Two showed how these loops take hold through repetition, like trails carved into a forest. But these trails aren't only cut by physical injury or movement. They're also widened and deepened by emotion and experience. And they can be significantly influenced by the constant background noise of life.

To understand why pain feels so overwhelming and hard to escape, we need to revisit the emotional brain. We will begin with the limbic system, which amplifies pain through the influence of fear and memory. Then we will discuss the prefrontal cortex, which interprets and assigns meaning. Then we will explore the roles of trauma, stress, and sensory overload, all of which teach the nervous system to stay on high alert. Together, these forces shape how pain is experienced. Not imagined, but literally shaped and magnified.

Revisiting the Brain's Pain Network

In Chapter One, we introduced the brain regions involved in processing pain. The thalamus acts as the relay station. Mapping falls on the somatosensory cortex. The limbic system and prefrontal cortex add emotional and cognitive layers to the brain. Now we need to return to these structures, not just to review them, but to understand how they don't simply register pain. They amplify it, alter it, and in some cases, generate it when the emotional brain is dysregulated.

This isn't redundant. It's essential. Understanding *where* pain is processed reveals what's happening, and understanding *how* emotion, memory, and interpretation shape that processing can explain *why* it feels the way it does. And more importantly, what you can do about it.

The Periaqueductal Gray: Pain's Volume Control

Before we dive into the emotional circuitry, there's one more structure worth understanding: the periaqueductal gray (PAG), located in the midbrain. The PAG is your brain's natural pain relief system.[1] It sends descending signals down the spinal cord that dampen incoming pain signals before they ever reach conscious awareness. This is how, in moments of extreme stress or danger, people can sustain injuries and feel little to no pain until the threat has passed.

But here's the problem. Chronic stress, trauma, and emotional dysregulation all weaken the PAG's ability to function. When the system is stuck in high alert, descending inhibition fails. The volume knob stays cranked up. Pain signals that should be dampened flow freely, and the nervous system loses one of its most powerful tools for regulating pain.

Understanding the PAG helps explain why relaxation techniques, mindfulness, and nervous system regulation strategies are more than just "nice to have." They directly influence your brain's ability to modulate pain at a physiological level. We'll return to the PAG's role throughout this chapter, especially when we discuss stress and how it undermines the body's natural pain control.

Why This Matters

You don't need to memorize these names or draw a map of your brain. What you need to understand is this. Pain isn't processed in one spot. Instead, it's a conversation between multiple regions. And each adds layers of emotion, interpretation, and intensity. When these regions become sensitized and dysregulated, they become stuck in a state of threat. And they don't just register pain. They magnify it. Alter it. And sometimes create it where none should exist.

Let me be very clear here. I'm not suggesting that your way of thinking is to blame for your pain. In fact, it has little to do with your thoughts. Most of what we're discussing happens beneath conscious awareness. The amygdala fires in response to threats, and the hippocampus pulls up old pain memories. Signals are amplified with emotion by the limbic system, and the release of stress hormones weakens your brain's natural pain control. None of this requires your permission or conscious thought. These are automatic processes and learned responses that fire before you even register what's happening. Even the guarding and the hypervigilance are patterns that run in the background, conditioned into your nervous system through repetition. You didn't choose them, nor did your thinking cause them to be there. This isn't weakness, it's neuroplasticity. Your brain is doing exactly what it's designed to do: learn, adapt, and protect. The problem is that it's learned patterns that no longer serve you.

The Limbic System: Where Pain Meets Emotion

Now let's go deeper into the emotional circuitry, focusing on the regions that turn a simple pain signal into an overwhelming experience. The limbic system is the brain's emotional engine. It processes fear, anxiety, memory, and stress, and it plays a massive role in how pain is felt.[2] When pain arises, the limbic system doesn't just register it. It gives it meaning and shapes the intensity of that pain.[3]

This translates into a fear that the pain will never end. Frustration arises from being unable to do what you once could. Anxiety comes from what the pain means for your future.

These emotions aren't separate from the pain; they're woven into it.[4] The more the limbic system fires in response to pain, the more amplified the signal becomes.

That's why stress feels like gasoline on the fire. The same pain can feel sharper and harder to manage when you're anxious or overwhelmed.[5] This doesn't mean the pain is imaginary. It means the brain's emotional circuits are magnifying a signal that is already real. The more often pain is paired with fear or worry, the easier it becomes to associate the two. After a sufficient amount of time, it begins to feel automatic.[6]

Let's look at the key structures within the limbic system and how each contributes to the pain experience.

The Amygdala: Your Threat Detector

The amygdala is your brain's alarm system. And it doesn't just react to danger, it learns from it.[7] When you experience pain repeatedly, the amygdala becomes hypersensitive. Especially when this pain is paired with fear or helplessness, ordinary sensations are then interpreted as threats. A muscle twinge that would generally go unnoticed suddenly feels like an alarm bell. The amygdala fires, causing your body to tense up and pain to intensify. This isn't imagination. Your threat detection system is doing precisely what it was designed to do, but doing it too well.

The Hippocampus: Memory and Context

The hippocampus provides context and memory. It helps your brain distinguish between past and present.[8] "I hurt my back once" versus "I always hurt my back." When the hippocampus functions well, it can dampen fear by providing accurate context. But trauma and chronic stress, on top of persistent pain, all impair hippocampal function. The result is that your brain struggles to update old threat associations, and it keeps treating the present as if it were the dangerous past. In doing so, it keeps reinforcing pain patterns that should have faded long ago.

The Anterior Cingulate Cortex (ACC): Where Sensation Becomes Suffering

The ACC is where sensation becomes suffering. It doesn't just register that you're in pain; it also determines how much that pain matters. In other words, it determines the level of distress and disruption to your life.[9] Research consistently shows that the ACC lights up more intensely in people with chronic pain. This is especially the case when they feel hopeless or catastrophic about their symptoms. This region bridges the gap between "I notice this" and "I can't take this anymore." Understanding this helps explain why two people with identical injuries can report vastly different levels of suffering.

The Insula: Your Internal Monitor

The insula tracks your internal landscape, such as your heart rate, muscle tension, gut sensations, and the position of your limbs. This process, known as interoception, is how you recognize when you're hungry, tired, anxious, or in pain.[10] In chronic pain, the insula often becomes hypervigilant. It monitors the body obsessively. It starts interpreting everyday signals as threats and amplifies pain intensity. People with chronic pain frequently report feeling "too aware" of their bodies, as if every sensation demands immediate attention. This is the result of an overwhelming flood of internal noise caused by the insula's inability to filter properly.

How They Work Together

These structures don't work in isolation. Instead, they constantly feed off each other. The amygdala detects threat and triggers fear. The hippocampus retrieves memories of past pain, thus confirming the threat. The ACC amplifies the emotional weight of the experience.

Together, they create a feedback loop where pain and emotion reinforce each other, exacerbating both.

The Prefrontal Cortex: Interpretation and Meaning

The limbic system doesn't work alone. The prefrontal cortex shapes how we interpret what the limbic system amplifies. If the limbic system is the amplifier, the prefrontal cortex is the interpreter. It assesses the meaning of pain and predicts whether or not it will worsen. Then, it determines how much attention to give it.[11] What you consciously think about your pain is determined here, and your interpretation can completely reshape your experience.

Imagine a sharp twinge in your back. One interpretation might be catastrophic: "Something is seriously wrong. I'll be crippled." That reading sparks panic. This increases muscle tension and stress hormones, which all make the pain sharper.[12] Another interpretation might be: "That was a strain, but I know my body can recover." Same physical signal. However, the brain allows the body to settle rather than spiral into fear.

This difference explains why two people with similar injuries or diagnoses can report wildly different levels of suffering. And again, it isn't about toughness or weakness. It's about how their brains have been taught to frame the pain.

This is why pain education matters. When you understand that a sharp twinge doesn't always mean damage, the prefrontal cortex has new information to work with. The interpretation shifts. And often, so does the intensity. Framing can be reshaped. Practices like reframing thoughts, journaling, or simply noticing patterns without judgment all work because they give the prefrontal cortex a new role: to break the automatic story of danger and replace it with a story of possibility.[13]

The prefrontal cortex also plays a crucial role in attention. Where you place your attention shapes what you feel. You may be hypervigilant, constantly scanning your body for signs of pain. The prefrontal cortex will direct more resources to monitoring those signals. The pain becomes louder simply because you're paying more attention to it. However, when you're deeply engaged in an activity you enjoy, the prefrontal cortex can shift attention away from pain. This reduces its intensity without altering the underlying signal.

This isn't a distraction in the dismissive sense. It's attention allocation. And it's a powerful tool for managing chronic pain. By understanding this, you recognize that, with time and the right approach, these signals can be reshaped.

The Stress Response: From Protective to Destructive

When interpretation meets emotion, the body responds with its oldest survival mechanism: the stress response. Pain fuels anxiety. Anxiety fuels pain. The body then shifts into sympathetic dominance, also known as the fight-or-flight response. When this happens, the limbic system begins to fire.[14] The result is that muscles will tighten, breathing becomes shallow, and the entire system operates on high alert. Stress hormones like cortisol and adrenaline flood the body, designed for short bursts to support survival.[15]

In the short term, this response is protective. It helps you escape danger, fight off threats, or endure difficult situations. As your heart rate increases, blood flow redirects to major muscles. This is preparing you for fight-or-flight. Usually, pain sensitivity temporarily decreases so you can focus on survival. This is why people can sustain injuries in high-stress situations and not feel the pain until afterward. The PAG, your brain's natural pain-relief system, kicks in during acute stress, releasing endorphins and dampening pain signals to keep you functional.

But when stress becomes chronic, this protective system turns destructive.

When Stress Won't Shut Off

When stress is constant, hormones do not fully return to normal levels. This leads to a vicious cycle of symptom reinforcement.[16] Cortisol, in particular, becomes dysregulated. For the record, cortisol isn't inherently bad. It actually wakes you up in the morning and helps you respond to challenges. But when it's chronically elevated, it disrupts the natural rhythm. Morning cortisol stays low when you need energy. Evening cortisol stays high when you need rest.[17] The system that once protected you now works against you, trapped in a pattern it can't break without intervention.

Sleep becomes another casualty of this cycle. Chronic stress disrupts sleep architecture. It reduces deep, restorative sleep needed to function well and replaces it with light, fragmented sleep.[18] The next day, pain thresholds drop. Sensations that were manageable yesterday may feel sharper today. And because poor sleep elevates stress hormones, the cycle reinforces itself. This trains the nervous system to treat even minor sensations as threats. Over time, the brain learns to anticipate and respond to pain. It begins to produce it, amplifying signals that otherwise might have gone unnoticed.[19] We'll explore this relationship in depth in a later chapter dedicated to sleep and recovery. But for now, understand that sleep isn't just rest. It's when the nervous system recalibrates, allowing the pain alarm system to quiet down.

Chronic stress hormones not only disrupt sleep cycles but also weaken immune function and further lower the threshold for pain.[20] This is maladaptive neuroplasticity at work: the brain learning a protective habit so thoroughly that it becomes a problem in itself.[21] The same learning processes that once helped you survive now perpetuate the pain loop.

The PAG Under Siege

Remember the PAG, your brain's volume control for pain? Chronic stress weakens its ability to dampen pain signals. When your nervous system is stuck in fight-or-flight mode, the PAG's descending inhibition fails.

The volume control stops working, and the pain that should be manageable becomes overwhelming. Not because the injury got worse, but because your nervous system lost its ability to regulate.

This isn't about mindset or simply thinking positively versus negatively. It's not about blaming yourself for doing something wrong. Most of the time, you don't even realize it's happening. It's a conditioned response, the brain automatically interpreting signals through patterns it has already learned.[22]

Trauma and the Nervous System

If constant stress primes the system, trauma takes that priming and hardwires it more deeply. It doesn't matter if it comes from a single overwhelming event or a series of smaller blows. Even if it stems from early-life instability, trauma leaves the nervous system on guard.[23] The limbic system fires faster. The prefrontal cortex interprets signals through a filter of danger.

Research on Adverse Childhood Experiences (ACEs) has shown that early trauma (abuse, neglect, household dysfunction) significantly increases the risk of chronic pain conditions later in life.[24] The nervous system learns threat early, and that learning shapes how it responds to everything that follows.

Living in this heightened state lowers the threshold for pain.[25] Muscles begin to brace. Sleep becomes restless, and stress hormones linger too long. Over time, the system starts to associate ordinary events with threats. Things as simple as reaching for a seatbelt, walking into a crowded store, or preparing for a difficult conversation. Each of these cues can trigger protective tightening, amplifying the sensations that follow.

This doesn't mean trauma creates pain out of nothing. It means trauma teaches the nervous system to expect it.[26] I know, I keep repeating this, but that's a testament to how important I believe it is to understand this. And that expectation is powerful enough to keep patterns alive long after tissues have healed. Guarding becomes a habit. Trigger points become easier to activate. The brain's body map narrows around what feels safe to use. Repeated trauma rewires the nervous system into expecting threat. This is a clear example of maladaptive neuroplasticity at work.[27]

And trauma doesn't just affect the amygdala and hippocampus. It also impairs the prefrontal cortex's ability to regulate emotions and to reframe threats as responses rather than threats themselves. When you've experienced repeated trauma, your brain's threat detection system becomes hypersensitive, and its regulation system becomes underactive. The balance tips toward constant vigilance, and pain becomes one more signal that the world isn't safe.

This is one of the cruelest aspects of chronic pain. The very system meant to protect you becomes the source of suffering. But here's what trauma survivors need to understand. Learned patterns can be replaced. Predictable routines, steady breathing, supportive relationships, and gentle, graded movements all give the nervous system new experiences to work with.[28] The alarm response eases, and the system spends less time on patrol. The imprint won't vanish overnight. But you can rewrite it with patient repetition.

Reflection prompt

Think of a time when pain showed up after a stressful or overwhelming event. Did the fear or tension seem to intensify the sensation? Did your body tense up before the pain even started? Identifying this can shed light on how expectations shape experiences.

Safety and Threat Detection

The nervous system operates on a simple question: Am I safe? When the answer is consistently "no" (whether from trauma, chronic stress, or constant sensory bombardment), the system remains vigilant. Over time, this vigilance becomes the baseline. The body forgets what safe feels like.[29]

This concept, articulated by Stephen Porges in his Polyvagal Theory, explains why recovery isn't just about treating pain.[30] It's about teaching the nervous system to recognize safety again. That process takes time, patience, and (most importantly) consistent experiences that prove safety is real.

Porges describes three states of nervous system activation: social engagement (safe and connected), mobilization (fight-or-flight), and immobilization (freeze or shutdown). Chronic pain patients often get stuck in mobilization or immobilization, unable to downshift into the social engagement state where healing can occur. The limbic system stays on high alert, the prefrontal cortex remains in threat-scanning mode, and the body never gets the signal that it's okay to relax.

Social isolation compounds this problem. Many chronic pain patients withdraw from activities and environments that once brought joy. Sometimes they even withdraw from relationships. This withdrawal removes protective social buffers, which are the very experiences that signal safety to the nervous system. Without these cues, the system has no reason to downshift from high alert.[31] The pain persists not just because of tissue damage or neural sensitization, but because the environment itself reinforces threat.

Human connection, safe touch, predictable routines, and environments where you feel genuinely at ease all send powerful signals to the limbic system: "You're safe. You can rest." Over time, these signals begin to retrain the nervous system. The threat detection system can now relax and allow pain to ease.

Sensory Overload in Modern Life

Imagine if you were trying to focus on one voice in a crowded stadium. Every sound competes for attention, and important signals get drowned out in the noise. For a nervous system already primed for threat, this chaos makes pain feel even sharper. If trauma in any form exists in the past, it can flood you with sensory overload. Chronic pain often flares not because of injury, but because of too much input. Noise. Light. Screens. Deadlines. Crowded environments. All of it taxes the brain's ability to filter and prioritize.[32]

A healthy nervous system can usually sort the meaningful from the background noise. But in a sensitized system, the filter wears thin.[33] Pain signals, caught in the flood, feel louder and more intrusive than they otherwise would. A typical conversation feels overwhelming. A bright grocery store feels unbearable. What's happening isn't weakness. It's the nervous system misfiring due to excessive weight.

The insula and prefrontal cortex are responsible for filtering sensory input. These structures determine what is relevant and what can be ignored. When these regions are overwhelmed by chronic stress or sensitization, they lose that ability. Everything feels equally important. Everything demands attention. The nervous system can't distinguish between a genuine threat and background noise, so it treats everything as a potential problem.

Modern life only adds to this. Constant phone alerts. Endless to-do lists. Environments full of stimulation. The nervous system gets little chance to downshift.[34] For someone already sensitized by trauma or stress, overload magnifies the alteration. The circuits meant to filter and dampen become stuck on the notion that "everything matters, everything is a threat."

Examples are everywhere. Trying to manage work emails while cooking dinner, or being surrounded by constant noise in an open office. Another is scrolling between apps late at night, trying to quiet a racing mind with more input. Or not being able to tolerate the grocery store, not because of physical weakness, but because the fluorescent lights, refrigerator hum, crying child, and overhead music create a sensory storm your nervous system can't filter.

But overload isn't always about noise or screens. Sometimes it's relational, such as living with a partner who requires constant emotional management. One who functions more like a dependent than an equal, or possibly even cycles through instability or addiction. This absolutely keeps the nervous system in a state of perpetual alert. You're not just managing your own stress. You're managing theirs, anticipating their moods, compensating for their dysfunction, and often doing it while also parenting actual children. The house might even get quiet at times. But the nervous system never rests. It doesn't distinguish between a chaotic environment and an unstable relationship. Both signal threats. Both drain resources. Both amplify pain. And often, the toll doesn't become clear until the stressor is gone.

All of these overload the system, making pain more intrusive and more exhausting.

Reducing sensory load isn't about avoiding life; it's about managing it effectively. It's about giving your nervous system breathing room. You can seek out quiet spaces. Taking intentional breaks from screens and dimming the lighting also helps. Limiting multitasking can also help, as too many open loops can increase anxiety that can become a signal that sets off a flare-up. All of these allow the brain to reset its filtering capacity. Over time, this can reduce the baseline level of nervous system arousal, making pain less intrusive and more manageable. And while this is not a book on things such as depression and anxiety, nor am I an expert on these conditions, I wonder how much this entire system affects how those conditions express themselves as well.

Reshaping the Emotional Brain

Here's where there is hope. The same brain circuits that amplify pain can also learn to reduce it.[35] The nervous system is plastic. What it learned can be unlearned. And the tools for doing so are within reach.

Mindful breathing teaches the nervous system to shift from fight-or-flight to rest-and-digest. Guided relaxation techniques can help calm the limbic system's hypervigilance. You can help the prefrontal cortex reframe interpretations and challenge catastrophic thoughts simply by journaling. Graded exposure to feared movements shows the brain that the perceived threat isn't real. Supportive relationships provide the social safety cues that allow the nervous system to downshift from high alert.

None of these erases pain instantly. But they all give the nervous system a new association: calm instead of threat, possibility instead of panic.[36] With repetition, these associations start to loosen the bond between pain and fear. Just as muscles retrain with exercise, emotional responses can also retrain with practice.[37]

The system can shift, even with small steps at a time. The amygdala becomes less reactive, and the hippocampus begins to distinguish between past and present. The ACC's interpretation of suffering softens. The insula learns to filter internal signals without flagging every sensation as a threat. And the PAG, your brain's natural pain relief system, regains its ability to dampen signals.

This doesn't diminish your experience. It validates it. If your pain spikes under stress or after overload, it's not because you're weak. It's because your brain is doing exactly what it was designed to do. It will pair pain with threat to keep you alert.[38] But that pairing is not fixed. You can reshape it. The nervous system is plastic, and what it learned can be unlearned.[39]

Understanding the emotional brain (and how it interacts with trauma and overload) bridges the science of pain with the lived experience of suffering. When you know that your amygdala is hypersensitive, or that your hippocampus is stuck in old patterns, you're not learning excuses. Or when you know that your prefrontal cortex is overwhelmed, and that your PAG has lost its ability to dampen signals, you're learning targets. Each of these systems can be influenced, retrained, and gradually brought back into balance.

Pulling It Together

Pain isn't just physical. It is processed, interpreted, and magnified through cortical maps, looping pathways, and the emotional brain. Trauma and stress, as well as overload, can all layer onto those systems, making pain louder, stranger, and much harder to escape.

However, they also point the way forward. As we have repeatedly stated, if pain is learned, it can be reshaped. And that possibility is what gives weight to everything that follows.

Reflection prompt

What environments or situations make you feel tense before pain even begins? How do those settings affect the way your body reacts? Bringing awareness to these triggers is the first step in changing them.

Common Myths That Keep People Stuck

Before we move forward, let's address a few common misconceptions that can often hinder you. These myths are everywhere: in doctors' offices, online forums, even in your own head. The more you can recognize them, the less power they have over you.

Myth: Pain always means damage.

Reality: Pain is a signal, but it can misfire. Your nervous system can become stuck, sending out alarm bells even when there's nothing left to protect.

Myth: If the scan is normal, the pain isn't real.

Reality: Most chronic pain doesn't show up on imaging. X-rays and MRIs show the structure, not how your nervous system processes signals.

Myth: Chronic pain is a mental health problem.

Reality: It's a nervous system problem, not a character flaw. Your brain isn't imagining the pain. It's amplifying and misinterpreting real signals.

Myth: You just need to push through it.

Reality: Pushing through can reinforce the pain loop. Your nervous system needs recalibration, not willpower.

Myth: If treatments haven't worked, nothing will.

Reality: Most people have tried the wrong treatments, not all treatments. The key is understanding why the pain persists, not just masking it.

These myths don't just live in your head. They're baked into how we talk about pain, how doctors are trained, and how society judges chronic illness. Recognizing them is the first step toward breaking free.

In the next section, we'll see how these mechanisms play out in specific conditions, such as Fibromyalgia, where the brain's filter breaks down entirely. We will also examine Ehlers-Danlos syndrome, which is characterized by a failure of proprioception that renders the body map unreliable. CRPS, where a minor injury triggers a cascade that the nervous system can't shut off. Each condition has its own story, but the root (maladaptive plasticity, emotional amplification, and learned threat responses) remains the same.

Endnotes

[1] Basbaum, A. I., & Fields, H. L. (1984). Endogenous pain control systems: brainstem spinal pathways and endorphin circuitry. *Annual Review of Neuroscience*, 7, 309-338.

[2] Bushnell, M. C., Čeko, M., & Low, L. A. (2013). Cognitive and emotional control of pain and its disruption in chronic pain. *Nature Reviews Neuroscience*, 14(7), 502-511.

[3] Wiech, K., & Tracey, I. (2013). Pain, decisions, and actions: a motivational perspective. *Frontiers in Neuroscience*, 7, 46.

[4] Apkarian, A. V., Baliki, M. N., & Farmer, M. A. (2013). Predicting transition to chronic pain. *Current Opinion in Neurology*, 26(4), 360-367.

[5] Edwards, R. R., Dworkin, R. H., Sullivan, M. D., Turk, D. C., & Wasan, A. D. (2016). The role of psychosocial processes in the development and maintenance of chronic pain. *The Journal of Pain*, 17(9), T70-T92.

[6] Vlaeyen, J. W., & Linton, S. J. (2000). Fear-avoidance and its consequences in chronic musculoskeletal pain: a state of the art. *Pain*, 85(3), 317-332.

[7] LeDoux, J. E. (2000). Emotion circuits in the brain. *Annual Review of Neuroscience*, 23, 155-184.

[8] Squire, L. R., & Zola, S. M. (1996). Structure and function of declarative and nondeclarative memory systems. *Proceedings of the National Academy of Sciences*, 93(24), 13515-13522.

[9] Rainville, P., Duncan, G. H., Price, D. D., Carrier, B., & Bushnell, M. C. (1997). Pain affect encoded in human anterior cingulate but not somatosensory cortex. *Science*, 277(5328), 968-971.

[10] Craig, A. D. (2009). How do you feel now? The anterior insula and human awareness. *Nature Reviews Neuroscience*, 10(1), 59-70.

[11] Lorenz, J., Minoshima, S., & Casey, K. L. (2003). Keeping pain out of mind: the role of the dorsolateral prefrontal cortex in pain modulation. *Brain*, 126(5), 1079-1091.

[12] Sullivan, M. J., Thorn, B., Haythornthwaite, J. A., Keefe, F., Martin, M., Bradley, L. A., & Lefebvre, J. C. (2001). Theoretical perspectives on the relation between catastrophizing and pain. *The Clinical Journal of Pain*, 17(1), 52-64.

[13] Dahl, J., Wilson, K. G., & Nilsson, A. (2004). Acceptance and commitment therapy and the treatment of persons at risk for long-term disability resulting from stress and pain symptoms: a preliminary randomized trial. *Behavior Therapy*, 35(4), 785-801.

[14] Porges, S. W. (2011). *The Polyvagal Theory: Neurophysiological Foundations of Emotions, Attachment, Communication, and Self-Regulation*. W. W. Norton & Company.

[15] Hannibal, K. E., & Bishop, M. D. (2014). Chronic stress, cortisol dysfunction, and pain: a psychoneuroendocrine rationale for stress management in pain rehabilitation. *Physical Therapy*, 94(12), 1816-1825.

[16] Finan, P. H., Goodin, B. R., & Smith, M. T. (2013). The association of sleep and pain: an update and a path forward. *The Journal of Pain*, 14(12), 1539-1552.

[17] McEwen, B. S., & Kalia, M. (2010). The role of corticosteroids and stress in chronic pain conditions. *Metabolism*, 59, S9-S15.

[18] Haack, M., Simpson, N., Sethna, N., Kaur, S., & Mullington, J. (2020). Sleep deficiency and chronic pain: potential underlying mechanisms and clinical implications. *Neuropsychopharmacology*, 45(1), 205-216.

[19] Nijs, J., Meeus, M., Versijpt, J., Moens, M., Bos, I., Knaepen, K., & Meeusen, R. (2015). Brain-derived neurotrophic factor as a driving force behind neuroplasticity in neuropathic and central sensitization pain: a new therapeutic target? *Expert Opinion on Therapeutic Targets*, 19(4), 565-576.

[20] Born, J., Lange, T., Hansen, K., Mölle, M., & Fehm, H. L. (1997). Effects of sleep and circadian rhythm on human circulating immune cells. *Journal of Immunology*, 158(9), 4454-4464.

[21] Woolf, C. J. (2011). Central sensitization: implications for the diagnosis and treatment of pain. *Pain*, 152(3), S2-S15.

[22] Moseley, G. L., & Vlaeyen, J. W. (2015). Beyond nociception: the imprecision hypothesis of chronic pain. *Pain*, 156(1), 35-38.

[23] van der Kolk, B. A. (2014). *The Body Keeps the Score: Brain, Mind, and Body in the Healing of Trauma.* Viking.

[24] Felitti, V. J., Anda, R. F., Nordenberg, D., Williamson, D. F., Spitz, A. M., Edwards, V., Koss, M. P., & Marks, J. S. (1998). Relationship of childhood abuse and household dysfunction to many of the leading causes of death in adults: The Adverse Childhood Experiences (ACE) Study. *American Journal of Preventive Medicine*, 14(4), 245-258.

[25] Afari, N., Ahumada, S. M., Wright, L. J., Mostoufi, S., Golnari, G., Reis, V., & Cuneo, J. G. (2014). Psychological trauma and functional somatic syndromes: a systematic review and meta-analysis. *Psychosomatic Medicine*, 76(1), 2-11.

[26] Gatchel, R. J., Peng, Y. B., Peters, M. L., Fuchs, P. N., & Turk, D. C. (2007). The biopsychosocial approach to chronic pain: scientific advances and future directions. *Psychological Bulletin*, 133(4), 581-624.

[27] Flor, H. (2003). *Cortical reorganisation and chronic pain: implications for rehabilitation.* Journal of Rehabilitation Medicine, 41(Suppl.), 66–72.

[28] Williams, A. C. D. C., Fisher, E., Hearn, L., & Eccleston, C. (2020). Psychological therapies for the management of chronic pain (excluding headache) in adults. *Cochrane Database of Systematic Reviews*, 8, CD007407.

[29] Kozlowska, K., Walker, P., McLean, L., & Carrive, P. (2015). Fear and the defense cascade: clinical implications and management. *Harvard Review of Psychiatry*, 23(4), 263-287.

[30] Porges, S. W. (2011). *The Polyvagal Theory: Neurophysiological Foundations of Emotions, Attachment, Communication, and Self-Regulation*. W. W. Norton & Company.

[31] Eisenberger, N. I., & Cole, S. W. (2012). Social neuroscience and health: neurophysiological mechanisms linking social ties with physical health. *Nature Neuroscience*, 15(5), 669-674.

[32] Nijs, J., Van Oosterwijck, J., De Hertogh, W., & Meeus, M. (2010). Scientific insights into chronic widespread pain and fatigue: the role of central sensitization and stress. Current Rheumatology Reviews, 6(3), 182–187

[33] Sarlani, E., & Greenspan, J. D. (2005). Why look in the brain for answers to temporomandibular disorder pain? *Cells Tissues Organs*, 180(1), 69-75.

[34] McEwen, B. S. (2006). Sleep deprivation as a neurobiologic and physiologic stressor: Allostasis and allostatic load. Sleep, 29(9), 1149–1155.

[35] Zeidan, F., Adler-Neal, A. L., Wells, R. E., Stagnaro, E., May, L. M., Eisenach, J. C., McHaffie, J. G., & Coghill, R. C. (2016). Mindfulness-meditation-based pain relief is not mediated by endogenous opioids. *The Journal of Neuroscience*, 36(11), 3391-3397.

[36] Kabat-Zinn, J. (2013). *Full Catastrophe Living: Using the Wisdom of Your Body and Mind to Face Stress, Pain, and Illness* (Revised edition). Bantam.

[37] Louw, A., Zimney, K., Puentedura, E. J., & Diener, I. (2016). The efficacy of pain neuroscience education on musculoskeletal pain: a systematic review of the literature. *Physiotherapy Theory and Practice*, 32(5), 332-355.

[38] Crombez, G., Eccleston, C., Van Damme, S., Vlaeyen, J. W., & Karoly, P. (2012). Fear-avoidance model of chronic pain: the next generation. *The Clinical Journal of Pain*, 28(6), 475-483.

[39] Moseley, G. L. (2004). *Evidence for a direct relationship between cognitive and physical change during an education intervention in chronic low back pain patients.* Pain, 108(1–2), 192–198.

Chapter 4

Fibromyalgia

A Nervous System in Overdrive

Before we begin, an important caveat: I am not suggesting that fibromyalgia, or any other condition discussed in this section, is caused exclusively by maladaptive neuroplasticity. These are complex conditions with many variables, and reducing them to a single mechanism would be both inaccurate and dismissive. What I am saying is that many of the strange, seemingly inexplicable ways these conditions express themselves don't fit neatly into diagnostic boxes. These symptoms, despite scans that come back normal and lead doctors to dismiss you, begin to make sense when viewed through the lens of maladaptive neuroplasticity. It is one common mechanism that often ties these conditions together, helping explain why they behave the way they do and why they've been so hard to understand.

One more note before we begin: This chapter, as well as the other chapters in the second section, is not meant to be a comprehensive guide to fibromyalgia or any of the other conditions referenced. My goal is to demonstrate how maladaptive neuroplasticity helps explain the unusual, seemingly random ways this condition manifests itself. I'm offering a lens, not the entire picture. Each condition discussed in this section deserves its own in-depth examination, and each intervention in Section Three has layers that we can't fully explore here. For this reason, I've included a Recommended Reading section at the end of this book, immediately preceding the bibliography. There, you'll find books and resources that delve deeper into fibromyalgia, Ehlers-Danlos syndrome, CRPS, and the various interventions we discuss. Think of this book as the map. Those resources are the territory.

With that foundation, let's talk about fibromyalgia.

In Chapter 3, we saw how emotion, trauma, and sensory overload amplify pain through the limbic system and stress responses. Now, in Section Two, we will apply that understanding to specific conditions. Fibromyalgia is the first. Not because it follows different rules, but because it shows what happens when those exact mechanisms are pushed to their extreme.[1] In the chapters that follow, we'll see other conditions (like Ehlers-Danlos or CRPS) expressing the same mechanisms in different ways.

Fibromyalgia has often been treated as an outlier. Patients are told it's mysterious, that it doesn't make sense, or worse, that it's all in their heads. Too often, when practitioners don't have a framework to explain what's happening, they default to dismissal. But fibromyalgia is not outside the rules of science. It's an extension of the same mechanisms of chronic pain we've already discussed, pushed into overdrive by the nervous system's own plasticity.[2]

Fibromyalgia can best be understood as a neuroplastic disorder.[3] The nervous system has learned to misinterpret and amplify signals, strengthening those pathways until pain feels louder, stranger, and more widespread than it should. This doesn't make the pain imaginary. It makes it learned. And what seems to be becoming a mantra in this book, what is learned can, with the right input, be relearned.[4]

What Fibro Patients Are Often Told

Before we dive into the mechanisms, it's worth acknowledging what many fibromyalgia patients hear when they seek help. You've probably been told some version of the following:

"Your tests came back normal."

"There's nothing physically wrong."

"Have you tried yoga? Maybe you're just stressed."

"It's probably just depression."

These responses aren't malicious. They're what happens when practitioners don't have a framework to explain what's in front of them. When imaging reveals no structural damage, and the pain doesn't follow a predictable pattern, the default is often dismissal. But normal test results don't mean imaginary pain. They tell us the problem isn't where we've been looking. The breakdown isn't in the tissues. It's in how the nervous system processes and interprets signals from those tissues.

Understanding fibromyalgia through the lens of neuroplasticity offers a different perspective. One that's grounded in science, that validates your experience, and that opens the door to meaningful intervention.

Cortical Maps and Strange Referrals

In Chapter 1, we discussed how the brain maintains dynamic cortical maps. In other words, internal representations of where your body is and what it's feeling. These maps are constantly updated based on sensory input, allowing you to localize sensation and move with precision. In fibromyalgia, these maps become profoundly altered.[5] The input is real, but the way it's amplified or misinterpreted creates an experience that feels overwhelming.[6]

This is where fibromyalgia diverges from typical chronic pain patterns. Remember the trigger point charts we discussed in Chapter 1? Those charts document referral patterns that occur in most people. These patterns have been mapped out over decades of observation and research. A trigger point in the upper trapezius sends pain into the head and behind the eye. A point in the glutes refers down the leg. These patterns are predictable and follow anatomical logic in about 75-80% of the population.

But in fibromyalgia, those patterns break down completely.

The brain's cortical maps become so altered that signals no longer follow predictable pathways. A trigger point in the shoulder might refer pain to the opposite hip. Pressure on the lower back might be felt as tingling in the jaw. These aren't the referrals you'd see on any chart. They don't follow nerve pathways. They don't respect anatomical boundaries. And they certainly don't make sense to anyone trying to explain them using traditional models.

Let me give you a real example. I had a patient who, when I pressed on her right hip flexor, felt sharp pain shoot into her left jaw. Not down the leg, not into the lower back, not where it's "supposed to refer." No, the referral went across the body and up into the face. According to traditional trigger point charts, this makes no sense. But through the lens of cortical remapping, we understand that the brain rerouted the pathway, thus creating a detour when the original map became too noisy to navigate.

Think of it like a city where construction has closed major highways. Drivers find workarounds, using side streets and back roads to get where they need to go. Those routes technically work, after all, they get you from point A to point B. But they don't make sense to anyone looking at a normal map. You're going three blocks out of your way, doubling back, cutting through neighborhoods that have nothing to do with your destination. To an outsider, it looks chaotic. But to the driver, it's the only way through.

Fibromyalgia works the same way. The brain's original pathways for processing sensation have become unreliable, so it reroutes. It finds new connections and develops new ways to interpret input. But those new routes don't follow the old logic. They're improvised. And because they're improvised, they shift.

This explains why fibro patients often describe their pain as migratory, widespread, and disconnected from any apparent injury.[7] You might wake with pain in your legs one morning, only for it to drift to your jaw or shoulders by evening. To you, it feels unpredictable and chaotic. You start to question whether it's real, whether you're imagining it, whether maybe the doctors are right and it's all in your head.

And technically, it is. But not in the way that dismissive phrase implies. It's in your brain's cortical maps. Every time pain shows up, the brain tries to organize it. It looks for patterns, a reason for it, and a place to file the information. But because the input is noisy and the maps are already altered, it ends up reinforcing the wrong connections. The detour becomes the new route. And then the detour changes again.

For example, pain may start in your neck after a car accident. Within six months, it spreads to your hips. A year later, your hands hurt constantly. You try physical therapy, massage, and acupuncture, but nothing sticks. But when you map your progression, the pattern becomes clear. An initial injury triggers central sensitization, which, over time, generalizes across the entire nervous system. The pain isn't spreading because tissue is failing in multiple locations. It spreads because your brain's map is being redrawn, region by region, as the nervous system learns to interpret more and more input as threat.

And it's not just about the location of the pain. The quality can shift, too. One moment it's sharp. The next, it's dull and achy. Then it burns, then tingles. This variability isn't due to the tissue changing. It's because the brain is interpreting the same noisy input in different ways, trying different explanations until it finds one that makes sense.

This also explains why fibro patients often feel dismissed when they try to describe their symptoms. A doctor asks, "Where does it hurt?" and you say, "My shoulder." The next visit, you say, "My hip." The visit after that, "My jaw." To the doctor, it looks inconsistent, maybe even fabricated. But what's actually happening is that your brain's map is unstable, and the pain is following the detours as they shift and reorganize.

Understanding this is critical because it shifts the conversation. Instead of asking, "Why doesn't this make sense?" we can ask, "What is my nervous system trying to tell me?" Instead of dismissing the pain as random, we can recognize it as the output of a system doing its best with faulty information. The pain is real. The referrals are real. But it's not chaos. It's an altered map trying to interpret a world that no longer matches its expectations.

Nerve Sprouting and the Noisy Signal

Cortical map alterations explain much of fibromyalgia's strangeness, but the chaos doesn't end in the brain. The peripheral nervous system compounds the problem. As we discussed in Chapter 1, peripheral nerves can sprout new branches after injury, attempting to restore function.[8] In fibromyalgia, this sprouting often backfires. Instead of creating clean, efficient pathways, the new branches overlap and misroute signals. This ends up flooding an already sensitized system with noisy input.[9]

Like we discussed in a previous analogy, picture trying to tune in to a radio station. When you're on the right frequency, the signal is clear. But move one notch off, and you start picking up fragments of the station mixed with static and interference from adjacent channels. The music is still there, but it's buried in noise. Nerve sprouting in fibromyalgia creates these overlapping signals that the brain struggles to parse.

This is why gentle touch can feel painful in fibro, or why clothing can become unbearable.[10] A nerve that used to report information only from your arm has now sprouted extra branches that overlap with neighboring regions, like the shoulder or upper back. When something touches your arm, the signal doesn't just say "touch on arm." It says, "touch on arm, and maybe shoulder, and maybe upper back too." The central nervous system, already sensitized and struggling to filter input, must now interpret this flood of overlapping signals. Instead of restoring balance, the system learns patterns that increase distress.

And because the nervous system is plastic, meaning it adapts to repeated input, these confusing messages get reinforced. The more often the brain receives the message "arm touch equals shoulder pain," the stronger that connection becomes. It's not a choice. It's not something you can will away. It's the nervous system doing what it's designed to do: learning from experience. The problem is, it's learning the wrong lessons.

Sprouting also doesn't happen in isolation. It feeds directly into the cortical map alterations we just discussed. Noisy peripheral input reaches an already amplified central system. The brain tries to organize the chaos, only to amplify it further. Together, these processes create a feedback loop where structural changes at the nerve level and functional changes in the brain reinforce each other, compounding the problem with each cycle.

What Breaks Down in Fibromyalgia

Now that we've seen how cortical maps and nerve sprouting create signal confusion, let's examine the broader systems that fail when fibromyalgia takes hold. These breakdowns occur at multiple levels, and each worsens the others.

Fibromyalgia brings together several breakdowns in pain processing that can exist individually in chronic pain. But in fibro, they stack on top of one another and compound. To better organize these issues, we'll examine them in two categories: neural breakdowns and systemic breakdowns. It is important to realize that these are not entirely distinct. Instead, they represent overlapping failures within a system struggling to maintain stability.

Neural Breakdowns

Let's start with what's happening in the nervous system itself.

Central Sensitization: The Volume Knob Stuck on High

As we explored in Chapter 2, central sensitization occurs when the nervous system becomes hypersensitive, amplifying normal or even mild sensations into painful ones. In fibromyalgia, this amplification is extreme.[11] The "volume knob" isn't just turned up; it's maxed out, and the dial has broken off.

Neuroimaging studies confirm this. When researchers subject fibro patients and healthy controls to the same pain stimulus by applying measured pressure to a specific body part, fibro patients exhibit significantly more activity in pain-processing regions of the brain.[12] Same input, wildly different response. This isn't about pain tolerance or toughness. It's about a nervous system that's interpreting normal input as a threat.

Imagine walking into a room where someone's music is turned up so loud you can't think. That's what the fibro nervous system is doing with every sensation. Light

111

touch feels like pressure. Pressure feels like pain. And pain feels unbearable. The amplification isn't a choice. It's a wiring problem.

Cortical Remapping: The Altered Map

The cortical map alterations we discussed earlier fall under this category. As the brain's sensory representations become amplified and reorganized, they no longer match the body's actual structure.[13] Signals get misrouted. Pain shows up in unexpected places. The system loses its ability to localize and interpret sensation accurately, creating the widespread, migratory pain that defines fibromyalgia.

Research using functional MRI shows that fibro patients have altered connectivity patterns in the somatosensory cortex and other pain-processing regions.[14] The brain's pain network becomes hyperconnected, meaning signals that should stay contained instead spread and amplify across multiple regions. This explains why a localized trigger can create body-wide symptoms.

Faulty Inhibitory Pathways: The Broken Brakes

Normally, the brain has descending circuits that act as brakes, dampening pain signals before they become overwhelming. These pathways, which we discussed in Chapter 1, send signals from the brain down the spinal cord, telling the pain system to quiet down. In fibromyalgia, those brakes don't work properly.[15]

Imagine trying to drive with worn-out brake pads. You press the pedal, but the car doesn't slow down the way it should. You push harder, and it slows a little, but it's not enough. Eventually, you realize you're just riding momentum, hoping you don't crash. That's what the fibro nervous system is doing. The brakes are there, technically. They don't engage the way they're supposed to.

This loss of inhibition is one of the reasons fibro pain feels so relentless. There's no off switch. Even when the initial input fades, the pain keeps firing because the system doesn't have a way to quiet itself. The amplification stays stuck, and without functional brakes, there's nothing to bring it back down.

Systemic Breakdowns

Now let's look at what's happening beyond the nervous system itself, in the body's broader regulatory systems.

Stress and Trauma Priming: The System on High Alert

In Chapter 3, we explored how trauma and chronic stress rewire the nervous system, priming the limbic system for hypervigilance and lowering pain thresholds. Many fibro patients have histories of trauma or prolonged stress.[16] This doesn't mean fibro is "psychological." It means their nervous system was conditioned to expect a threat, and that conditioning makes the system more vulnerable to sensitization.

When you live in a state of chronic stress, your body produces elevated levels of cortisol, the primary stress hormone. Cortisol is helpful in short bursts as it helps you respond to danger. But when it remains elevated for weeks, months, or years, it begins to erode the system. Sleep gets disrupted. Vigilance becomes the default. And the threshold for pain drops lower and lower.

The nervous system learns to interpret everything as potentially dangerous because, for a long time, that was the safest assumption. Even after the stressor is gone, the pattern remains. The brain has been conditioned to expect the worst, and it continues to act accordingly.

It's not that trauma causes fibro. It's that trauma sets the stage for it. It lowers the threshold, primes the system, and makes it easier for pain to take hold. And once it does, the loop reinforces itself.

Sleep and Recovery Disruption: The System That Never Resets

As we discussed in Chapter 2, the pain loop is a self-reinforcing cycle: pain disrupts sleep, poor sleep amplifies pain, and the cycle deepens. Fibromyalgia patients live this loop daily. Poor sleep quality is nearly universal among those with the condition.[17]

This isn't just "I didn't sleep well last night" fatigue. This is waking up exhausted, feeling like you never slept at all. Even if you got eight or nine hours in bed. Many patients describe it as feeling like they were hit by a truck overnight.

Without restorative sleep, the nervous system doesn't reset properly. Think of sleep as the brain's maintenance window. It's when the system clears out metabolic waste, consolidates memories, and recalibrates pain thresholds. When that process gets interrupted night after night, the system starts to fall apart.

Fatigue, combined with sensitization, makes the system even more reactive. Pain lowers the quality of sleep, and poor sleep intensifies pain. It's a vicious cycle, and breaking out of it is one of the most challenging aspects of managing fibromyalgia.

Autonomic Nervous System Dysregulation: Stuck in Fight-or-Flight

Remember in Chapter 3, we discussed how the autonomic nervous system regulates unconscious functions such as heart rate, blood pressure, and digestion. The result is oscillation between sympathetic (fight-or-flight) and parasympathetic (rest-and-digest) states. Research indicates that many fibromyalgia patients experience altered autonomic balance, characterized by excessive sympathetic activity and inadequate parasympathetic tone.[18] The sympathetic nervous system is your "fight or flight" mode. It's designed to activate in emergencies and then deactivate. The parasympathetic system is where you recover, calm down, and restore.

In fibro, the sympathetic system stays stuck in the "on" position. The body remains in a state of high alert, with little access to its restorative systems. This imbalance explains many of the non-pain symptoms that fibromyalgia patients experience: dizziness, digestive problems, changes in heart rate, and intolerance to stress or temperature changes. The body is running on overdrive, burning fuel it doesn't have, and never getting a chance to recover.

It's exhausting. Not just physically, but systemically. Every system in the body is constantly being asked to function at maximum capacity, with no breaks.

Immune and Glial Involvement: The Silent Inflammation

Emerging studies suggest that low-grade neuroinflammation, glial cell activation, and altered cytokine signaling may contribute to the persistence of fibromyalgia.[19] Glial cells are the support cells in the nervous system. They're supposed to help neurons function, provide nutrients, and remove debris. But in fibro, they seem to become overprotective. They flood the system with signals that keep pain circuits firing, even when there's no real threat.

Think of them as neighbors who want to help but won't stop knocking on the door. Their intentions are good. But the constant interruption makes it impossible to rest. This neuroinflammation isn't the type that would show up on a blood test. It's subtle, often localized, and very difficult to measure. But it's real, and it's contributing to the noise.

How They Feed Each Other

Here's the thing. Each of these mechanisms worsens the others. Sensitization makes sleep harder. Poor sleep intensifies sensitization. Trauma primes both. Autonomic imbalance keeps the body on alert, making it harder to sleep. This worsens pain and increases stress. The immune system reacts to the stress, fueling further inflammation. This, in turn, keeps glial cells active and maintains the pain circuits.

It's not chaos. It's a feedback loop. And once it gets going, it's tough to stop.

This is why fibromyalgia appears so confusing to outside observers. Doctors see normal test results and assume there's nothing wrong. But the breakdown isn't in the tissues. It's in how the systems communicate with each other. The wiring is intact, but the signals are all wrong. The volume is too loud. The brakes don't work. The maintenance window is closed, and the entire system is running on fumes.

Understanding this won't make the pain go away. But it can help make sense of it. And that's the first step in figuring out how to intervene.

Beyond Pain: The Cognitive and Systemic Toll

Fibromyalgia doesn't stop at pain. One of the most debilitating aspects is cognitive dysfunction, often described as "fibro fog." Patients report memory lapses, difficulty concentrating, and slowed thinking.[20] This isn't imaginary. It reflects how much of the brain's resources are dedicated to interpreting and responding to amplified pain signals.

Think of your brain like a computer with limited processing power. When too many programs are running at once, everything slows down. The cursor lags. Applications freeze. Basic tasks that should take seconds now take minutes. You're not doing anything wrong. The system is just overloaded.

Fibro fog feels the same way. When pain dominates, it doesn't just hurt; it demands attention. The brain must monitor, interpret, respond to, and make sense of it. All of that takes energy. All of that uses bandwidth. And when most of your brain's resources are devoted to managing pain, there's less left over for everything else, like clear thinking, memory, decision-making, and executive function.

The pain isn't just interrupting your day. It's occupying mental space that would otherwise be available for focus and clarity.

This is why fibro patients often describe feeling mentally exhausted even when they haven't done anything cognitively demanding. You sit down to read a paragraph and realize you have to read it three times before it sinks in. You walk into a room and forget why you went there. You're mid-sentence when you completely lose your train of thought.

It's not early-onset dementia. It's not you losing your mind. It's a brain running too many background processes, and something has to give.

The frustration this creates is real. You know you're capable of more. You remember what it felt like to think clearly and to hold multiple ideas in your head at once. You used to finish a task without constantly forgetting what you were doing. But now even simple conversations feel like they require too much effort. You're working twice as hard to do half as much. And nobody around you seems to understand why.

What makes it worse is that fibro fog isn't constant. Some days are clearer than others. You might have a morning when your mind feels sharp, but by afternoon, you're struggling to form coherent sentences. This variability makes it hard to predict and even harder to explain. And it makes it very easy for others to dismiss. If you can think clearly sometimes, why not all the time?

But that logic misses the point. The fog isn't about effort or willpower. It's about how much cognitive load the brain is carrying at any given moment. On a low-pain day, there's more bandwidth. On a high-pain day, there's less.

There's also the issue of sleep, because poor sleep compounds cognitive dysfunction. When you're not sleeping well, your brain doesn't get the chance to consolidate memories or clear out metabolic waste. The result is that even on days when pain is relatively manageable, your thinking still feels sluggish because the system hasn't had time to reset. Pain disrupts sleep. Sleep deprivation worsens pain and cognition. And round and round it goes.

Fibromyalgia also often overlaps with other conditions rooted in central sensitization, such as migraines, irritable bowel syndrome (IBS), temporomandibular joint disorder (TMJ), or interstitial cystitis.[21] These comorbidities aren't coincidental. They reinforce the idea that fibro is not a separate mystery illness but a systemic manifestation of nervous system hypersensitivity and maladaptive neuroplasticity.

Someone dealing with both IBS and fibro, for instance, is experiencing the same hypersensitivity expressed in different organ systems. The gut becomes overly reactive to normal digestive input, just as the musculoskeletal system becomes excessively reactive to normal movement or touch. The migraine brain amplifies sensory input (light, sound, smell) in the same way the fibro brain amplifies pain. The mechanisms are the same. The location is different.

This overlap is actually useful diagnostically. When you start seeing multiple conditions from the central sensitization family clustering together, it points to a shared root cause rather than a collection of unrelated problems. It's not that you're unlucky and happened to develop five different conditions. It's that your nervous system has become hypersensitive across the board, and this hypersensitivity is manifesting in various ways, depending on where the system is most vulnerable.

Understanding this can be both validating and overwhelming. Validating, because it confirms that what you're experiencing is real and has a physiological basis. But it can also be overwhelming because it means the problem isn't isolated to one area. It's systemic.

But being systemic also means there's potential for systemic intervention. If the root cause is nervous system dysregulation, then interventions that calm the nervous system can help across the board. You're not fighting five separate battles. You're addressing one underlying issue that's expressing itself in multiple ways.

The cognitive and systemic symptoms of fibromyalgia are often what push patients to the edge. Pain is hard enough. But when you add brain fog, fatigue, digestive issues, headaches, and a dozen other symptoms that don't fit neatly into a single diagnosis, it starts to feel unbearable. You feel like your body is betraying you in every possible way. And the worst part is, most of these symptoms are invisible. Nobody can see your brain fog. Nobody can measure your fatigue on a blood test. So even when you're struggling, you're expected to function as if everything is fine.

But it's not fine. And pretending it is only makes it worse. These symptoms matter. They're part of the picture. Addressing them requires the same approach as addressing the pain itself: recognizing that the nervous system is overwhelmed, providing it with the support it needs to recalibrate, and slowly rebuilding stability one small step at a time.

Why Fibro Makes Sense

When viewed through the lens of neuroplasticity and cortical mapping, fibromyalgia ceases to be an enigma and begins to make sense. The unusual referral patterns, the widespread distribution, and the unpredictability all follow from the same principles of maladaptive learning described in Section One.[22] Fibro isn't a separate disease carved out from the rest of medicine. It's a chronic pain state where the brain's map of the body has been altered, the volume knob has been turned up, and the system has lost its ability to filter and regulate input effectively.

For years, fibromyalgia has been treated like a puzzle with missing pieces. Doctors couldn't find structural damage. Lab work came back normal. Imaging didn't show anything wrong. The assumption was that nothing was wrong, that it was psychological, or that patients were exaggerating. But the pieces weren't missing. We were looking in the wrong place.

The problem isn't in the tissues. It's in how the nervous system interprets signals from those tissues. Once you understand that, everything else clicks into place. The shifting pain makes sense because the brain's maps are unstable. The hypersensitivity makes sense because the volume knob is stuck on high. The fatigue and brain fog make sense because the system is constantly running at maximum capacity with no chance to rest. Even the comorbidities make sense, because they're all expressions of the same underlying hypersensitivity.

This perspective also reshapes the narrative for patients. Instead of being told their condition is untreatable or meaningless, they can understand it as a system that has learned the wrong patterns that, with persistence and the right approaches, can be reshaped. And that's not just hopeful thinking. It's backed by research.

Understanding the mechanisms isn't just intellectually satisfying; it's also personally gratifying. It opens the door to interventions that target those exact pathways. If the problem is a sensitized nervous system, the solution is to teach that system to calm down. If the problem is faulty inhibitory pathways, the solution is to strengthen them. If the problem is altered cortical maps, the solution is to provide the brain with new, accurate information to work with.

Take exercise, for example. It's one of the most well-studied interventions for fibro, and it works.[23] But not because it "strengthens" damaged tissues or "fixes" structural problems. What it actually does is recalibrate sensory input. When you move in a controlled, gradual way, you're teaching the nervous system that movement is safe. You're feeding the brain new information: "This doesn't hurt. This is okay. You can tolerate this." Over time, the system starts to trust that input. The volume knob comes down, just a little. The hypersensitivity eases slightly.

A patient might begin with simple exercises such as chair squats or short walks. Five minutes. Ten minutes. Whatever feels manageable. The goal isn't to push through pain or prove toughness. The goal is to provide the nervous system with repeated exposure to safe movement, allowing it to begin relearning what normal feels like. Gradually, as the system adapts, you increase exposure. Not because you're getting stronger in the traditional sense, but because the brain is recalibrating its threat response.

Graded activity works the same way.[24] The idea is to prevent flare-ups while still feeding the brain new, safe experiences. You're not avoiding activity altogether. You're strategically pacing it, giving the system manageable doses of input so it doesn't get overwhelmed.

Cognitive-behavioral therapy (CBT) is another intervention with substantial evidence.[25] It helps shift interpretations of pain signals, reducing their emotional impact. CBT doesn't claim pain is imaginary. It recognizes that the way you think about pain influences how much it disrupts your life. If every pain flare sends you into panic ("This will never get better, I'm broken, I can't do anything"), that emotional response amplifies the pain signal. The limbic system lights up, stress hormones flood the system, and the pain gets worse.

CBT teaches you to notice those thoughts and reframe them. Not in a "just think positive" sort of way. But in a realistic, grounded way. "This is a flare. Flares happen. They pass. I've been through this before, and I'll get through it again." That shift doesn't erase the pain, but it takes some of the emotional fuel out of the fire. And when the emotional amplification comes down, the pain often follows.

Mindfulness practices work along similar lines.[26] They calm limbic over-activation and reduce stress-driven amplification. Simple routines like body scans or breathing exercises can help down-regulate the nervous system, shifting it out of fight-or-flight mode and into a calmer baseline. You're not meditating the pain away. You're giving the nervous system permission to stop treating everything as an emergency.

And then there's sleep. Improved sleep hygiene helps restore some of the reset mechanisms that lower sensitivity, allowing the nervous system to rest and recalibrate.[27] This is harder than it sounds, because pain disrupts sleep and poor sleep worsens pain. But even minor improvements matter. Darkening the room, maintaining a consistent bedtime, and avoiding screens for an hour before bed. These aren't cure-alls, but they give the system a slightly better chance to do what it's supposed to do overnight: clear metabolic waste, consolidate memory, and bring the volume back down.

None of these interventions cure fibro. Let's be honest about that. They don't erase the condition or rewind the clock to before it started. But they provide new inputs that help the nervous system recalibrate. Over time, those inputs accumulate. One less flare after exercise. A night of deeper sleep. An easier time concentrating. A moment where the pain didn't completely dominate your attention.

Small victories accumulate. The system starts to learn that not everything is a threat. The volume knob inches downward. The maps stabilize, just a little. The inhibitory pathways begin to engage more reliably. It's not a straight line. There are setbacks. There are days when it feels like nothing is working. But the trajectory can shift over time.

And that's the point. Fibromyalgia isn't a life sentence. It's a learned state. And what is learned can, with patience and persistence, be unlearned. Not completely. Not perfectly. But enough to reclaim function, reduce suffering, and start living again in ways that feel meaningful.

Fibro as a Neuroplastic Disorder

At its core, fibromyalgia is the nervous system responding under strain. It is maladaptive neuroplasticity: the same capacity to learn and adapt that makes humans resilient can also hardwire pain.[28]

That doesn't make fibro untreatable. It makes it plastic, and plastic systems can change.

The therapeutic tools remain the same: movement, manual therapy, sleep, stress reduction, and nervous system retraining are still the foundational building blocks. What changes is how they are applied. For fibro patients, the map is unique, so treatment must be tailored accordingly. But the principles remain the same. And importantly, effective care must address not only pain but the broader systemic picture: improving sleep, calming the autonomic system, supporting cognition, and reducing neuroinflammation.

That's the core message I want fibro patients to take away from this chapter. Your pain isn't random or meaningless. It's the nervous system doing what it always does, learning, adapting, and sometimes misfiring. And because it's based on neuroplasticity, it can change.[29] We may not be able to erase fibro, but we can redraw the map. With enough time, we can reduce the noise and reclaim function. That isn't false hope. It's the science of how the nervous system works.

As we move forward, we'll see that while fibromyalgia may be the clearest example of these processes, other conditions, such as Ehlers-Danlos or CRPS, reflect the same mechanisms in different ways. If fibro represents the system turned up to maximum, Ehlers-Danlos shows how structural instability creates a different but equally telling expression of the same nervous system story.

Reflection Prompt

It's helpful to pause here and consider your own experience. Think about a time when your pain shifted from one area to another without explanation. How did it affect your confidence in understanding your own body? And which of these breakdowns, sleep, stress, immune, or autonomic, do you recognize most in your own experience?

Bringing awareness to these patterns isn't about blame or judgment. It's the first step in understanding what your nervous system is doing, and why it might be doing it.

Endnotes

[1] Clauw, D. J. (2014). Fibromyalgia: A clinical review. *JAMA*, 311(15), 1547–1555.

[2] Woolf, C. J. (2011). Central sensitization: Implications for the diagnosis and treatment of pain. *Pain*, 152(3 Suppl), S2–S15.

[3] Moseley, G. L., & Flor, H. (2012). Targeting cortical representations in the treatment of chronic pain: A review. *Neurorehabilitation and Neural Repair*, 26(6), 646–652.

[4] Moseley, G. L., & Butler, D. S. (2015). Fifteen years of explaining pain: The past, present, and future. *Journal of Pain*, 16(9), 807–813.

[5] Flor, H. (2003). *Cortical reorganisation and chronic pain: implications for rehabilitation.* Journal of Rehabilitation Medicine, 41(Suppl.), 66–72.

[6] Pujol, J., López-Solà, M., Ortiz, H., et al. (2009). Mapping brain response to pain in fibromyalgia patients using temporal analysis of fMRI. *PLOS ONE*, 4(4), e5224.

[7] Moseley, G. L. (2003). A pain neuromatrix approach to patients with chronic pain. *Manual Therapy*, 8(3), 130–140.

[8] Woolf, C. J., & Ma, Q. (2007). Nociceptors—noxious stimulus detectors. *Neuron*, 55(3), 353–364.

[9] Oaklander, A. L., Herzog, Z. D., Downs, H. M., & Klein, M. M. (2013). Objective evidence that small-fiber polyneuropathy underlies some illnesses currently labeled as fibromyalgia. *Pain*, 154(11), 2310–2316.

[10] Geisser, M. E., Glass, J. M., Rajcevska, L. D., et al. (2008). A psychophysical study of auditory and pressure sensitivity in patients with fibromyalgia and healthy controls. *Journal of Pain*, 9(5), 417–422.

[11] Staud, R., Vierck, C. J., Cannon, R. L., Mauderli, A. P., & Price, D. D. (2001). Abnormal sensitization and temporal summation of second pain (wind-up) in patients with fibromyalgia syndrome. *Pain*, 91(1–2), 165–175.

[12] Cook, D. B., Lange, G., Ciccone, D. S., Liu, W. C., Steffener, J., & Natelson, B. H. (2004). Functional imaging of pain in patients with primary fibromyalgia. *Journal of Rheumatology*, 31(2), 364–378.

[13] Kim, J., Loggia, M. L., Cahalan, C. M., et al. (2015). The somatosensory link in fibromyalgia: Functional connectivity of the primary somatosensory cortex is altered by sustained pain and is associated with clinical/autonomic dysfunction. *Arthritis & Rheumatology*, 67(5), 1395–1405.

[14] Jensen, K. B., Loitoile, R., Kosek, E., et al. (2012). Patients with fibromyalgia display less functional connectivity in the brain's pain inhibitory network. Pain, 153(5), 1018–1026.

[15] Julien, N., Goffaux, P., Arsenault, P., & Marchand, S. (2005). Widespread pain in fibromyalgia is related to a deficit of endogenous pain inhibition. *Pain*, 114(1–2), 295–302.

[16] Häuser, W., Kosseva, M., Üceyler, N., Klose, P., & Sommer, C. (2011). Emotional, physical, and sexual abuse in fibromyalgia syndrome: A systematic review with meta-analysis. *Arthritis Care & Research*, 63(6), 808–820.

[17] Roehrs, T., & Roth, T. (2005). Sleep and pain: Interaction of two vital functions. *Seminars in Neurology*, 25(1), 106–116.

[18] Martínez-Lavín, M., Hermosillo, A. G., Rosas, M., & Soto, M. E. (1998). Circadian studies of autonomic nervous balance in patients with fibromyalgia: A heart rate variability analysis. *Arthritis & Rheumatism*, 41(11), 1966–1971.

[19] Albrecht, D. S., Forsberg, A., Sandström, A., et al. (2019). Brain glial activation in fibromyalgia: A multi-

site positron emission tomography investigation. *Brain, Behavior, and Immunity*, 75, 72–83.

[20] Glass, J. M. (2009). Review of cognitive dysfunction in fibromyalgia: A convergence on working memory and attentional control impairments. *Rheumatic Disease Clinics of North America*, 35(2), 299–311.

[21] Yunus, M. B. (2007). Fibromyalgia and overlapping disorders: The unifying concept of central sensitivity syndromes. *Seminars in Arthritis and Rheumatism*, 36(6), 339–356.

[22] Clauw, D. J. (2015). Diagnosing and treating chronic musculoskeletal pain based on the underlying mechanism(s). *Best Practice & Research Clinical Rheumatology*, 29(1), 6–19.

[23] Busch, A. J., Webber, S. C., Richards, R. S., et al. (2013). Resistance exercise training for fibromyalgia. *Cochrane Database of Systematic Reviews*, 12, CD010884.

[24] Nijs, J., Paul van Wilgen, C., Van Oosterwijck, J., van Ittersum, M., & Meeus, M. (2011). How to explain central sensitization to patients with 'unexplained' chronic musculoskeletal pain: Practice guidelines. *Manual Therapy*, 16(5), 413–418.

[25] Bernardy, K., Klose, P., Busch, A. J., Choy, E. H., & Häuser, W. (2013). Cognitive behavioural therapies for

fibromyalgia. *Cochrane Database of Systematic Reviews*, 9, CD009796.

[26] Lakhan, S. E., & Schofield, K. L. (2013). Mindfulness-based therapies in the treatment of somatization disorders: A systematic review and meta-analysis. *PLOS ONE*, 8(8), e71834.

[27] Tang, N. K., Goodchild, C. E., Sanborn, A. N., Howard, J., & Salkovskis, P. M. (2012). Deciphering the temporal link between pain and sleep in a heterogeneous chronic pain patient sample: A multilevel daily process study. *Sleep*, 35(5), 675–687.

[28] Flor, H. (2012). New developments in the understanding and management of persistent pain. *Current Opinion in Psychiatry*, 25(2), 109–113.

[29] Moseley, G. L., & Butler, D. S. (2015). Fifteen years of explaining pain: The past, present, and future. *Journal of Pain*, 16(9), 807–813.

Chapter Five

Ehlers Danlos Syndrome

When Structure Collapses

In Chapter 4, we discussed fibromyalgia and how it puts the nervous system in overdrive, and how it amplifies every signal until pain dominates the landscape. Ehlers–Danlos Syndrome (EDS) shows us the flip side of the coin. It's what happens when the body's structure collapses, flooding the nervous system with unreliable input that demands constant compensation. The mechanisms, maladaptive neuroplasticity, altered cortical maps, and nervous system dysregulation are all the same. But the entry point is different.

Most people's bodies hold themselves together without thought. Ligaments stabilize joints automatically. Muscles contract and release in rhythm. The body knows where it is in space, what it's doing, and how to move efficiently. For people with Ehlers–Danlos Syndrome, that's a full-time job. And the shift never ends.

Imagine waking up and feeling your shoulder slip slightly out of the socket as you reach for your phone. You adjust, carefully, and it slides back into place with a dull ache that will linger for hours. You stand, and your knee hyperextends backward just enough to send a jolt of pain up your thigh. By the time you've brushed your teeth and gotten dressed, you've already stabilized a dozen joints manually, braced against movements that should feel automatic, and made a mental calculation about how much energy you have left for the day. And the day has barely started.

This is the reality of living with EDS. Instead of hypersensitivity altering the map, EDS begins with connective tissue instability. Joints that move too far. Ligaments that fail to provide the support they're designed to give. Muscles forced to pick up the slack, guarding constantly, never quite able to rest. The result is pain, fatigue, and injury cycles that feed into the same maladaptive neuroplasticity described in earlier chapters. The rules don't change. The starting point does.

The Misunderstood Strength of Constant Compensation

Here's something most people don't understand about EDS. These patients are not weak. They may struggle with tasks that seem simple. But their muscles are often overdeveloped, hypertrophied from years of compensating for ligamentous laxity, not the other way around. The problem for them isn't a lack of strength. The problem is that their muscles never get to rest.

Imagine someone tells you to do bicep curls with two-pound weights. Easy. You'd barely feel it. Now imagine doing those curls from the moment you wake up in the morning, nonstop, until you fall asleep at night. And even then, finding a way to keep doing them while you sleep. Days, weeks, months. See how much things start to hurt. See how exhausted you become.

That's what EDS patients are living through. Their muscles are perpetually contracted, stabilizing joints that ligaments should stabilize. The tension never fully releases. There's no break, no recovery period. The muscles are working overtime, all the time. And the result is not strength but exhaustion. Pain. Dysfunction.

This is why EDS patients can sometimes even appear to be in shape despite profound fatigue and pain. They're not weak. They're overworked. Their bodies are running a marathon every single day just to maintain basic stability. And people who don't understand this see the muscle tone and assume the patient is fine, or exaggerating, or not trying hard enough. The truth is the opposite. They're trying too hard because their bodies give them no choice.

Living with this instability often means waking up already tired. It sometimes means not knowing if today will bring another dislocation, so you end up bracing yourself for tasks as small as carrying groceries or even climbing stairs. Patients sometimes even describe feeling like their bodies betray them. Joints slip out of place without warning, and pain arises unpredictably, unconnected to any apparent cause. Even sitting upright at a desk can feel exhausting, because the body is constantly working to hold itself together. Every movement requires stabilization that most people's ligaments provide automatically. For someone with EDS, every movement is a negotiation.

This instability leaves patients feeling vulnerable in ways hard to explain to those who haven't lived it. Every day life can feel unstable. It feels like you're walking on thin ice, and you never know when it will crack. Holding posture at a desk may feel like a workout, and something as simple as lifting a child or carrying laundry can trigger anxiety because the smallest twist might cause a joint to shift. Even social interactions can become draining. Not just because of physical fatigue, but because of the unpredictability.

The constant worry of "What if my body fails me here?" weighs on every decision.

The nervous system doesn't ignore this vulnerability. It adapts. And often, that adaptation comes at a cost.

Proprioception and the Fuzzy Map

One of the most distinctive aspects of EDS is how it disrupts proprioception, the brain's sense of where the body is in space.[1] Most people move through the world with an intuitive understanding of their limbs' position. You can reach for a cup without looking. You can walk across a dark room without stumbling. You know, without thinking, where your body ends, and the world begins. That internal map is constantly updated by signals from muscles, joints, and skin, all feeding information to the brain about position, tension, and movement.

In EDS, that map becomes blurred.[2] Ligaments that should provide clear feedback about joint position are too lax to send reliable signals. Muscles compensate by guarding excessively, but their feedback is altered by constant tension. The brain receives conflicting information. Is the joint stable or not? Or is this movement safe or risky? The signals don't match, resulting in proprioceptive lag. It's like driving with a GPS that gives directions two seconds late. You overshoot every turn, correct, veer back, and the whole drive feels wrong.

Many EDS patients describe it as clumsiness, frequent stumbles, or a sense of disconnection from their bodies. They may feel like they're moving through fog, never quite sure where their limbs are until they make contact with something. Or they end up overcompensating, bracing too hard, moving too carefully. So they end up exhausting themselves with vigilance.

This fuzzy mapping forces the nervous system to work harder to stabilize movements. Muscles try to provide stability that the ligaments cannot by tightening and guarding excessively. Over time, this guarding rewires cortical maps and reinforces pain pathways.[3] The more the brain has to correct for instability, the more it strengthens maladaptive patterns. Instead of efficiently interpreting signals, the nervous system falls into a loop of overcorrection and pain. What begins as structural instability becomes a learned cycle of fatigue and overprotection.

The Nervous System's Role

EDS creates a perfect storm for maladaptive neuroplasticity. Structural instability floods the nervous system with confusing proprioceptive input. The brain attempts to make sense of unreliable signals by reinforcing guarding patterns, which only deepen the dysfunction. Over time, these protective responses become the problem.[4]

This is what it looks like in practice. A person with EDS reaches for a book on a high shelf. The shoulder joint, lacking adequate ligamentous support, shifts slightly. The brain registers this shift as a threat, so muscles around the shoulder contract reflexively to prevent further movement. They retrieve the book and lower their arm, but the muscles don't fully release. Even though the "threat" has passed, they remain in spasm to guard against it. Over hours, days, weeks, this pattern repeats. The brain reinforces the guarding response. The shoulder becomes chronically tense. Pain sets in, not from the original instability, but from the constant muscular spasm designed to protect against it.

Now multiply that across every joint in the body. The neck guards against the head's weight on an unstable cervical spine. Or the hips, bracing against the instability of hypermobile sacroiliac joints. Ligamentous laxity in the ankles causes them to adjust and overcompensate constantly. The entire musculoskeletal system becomes a web of compensation, each guarded joint creating new stress on surrounding structures. And the nervous system, trying to manage all of this, becomes increasingly sensitized to any signal that might indicate instability.

This is why EDS patients often describe pain that doesn't make anatomical sense. A patient may have right hip pain that seems linked to tension in their left shoulder. The pain isn't following nerve pathways or dermatomes. It's following the body's compensatory patterns, the ways the nervous system has learned to distribute tension and guarding across multiple joints in an attempt to create stability where the connective tissue cannot.[5]

The Diagnostic Maze and Medical Dismissal

For many patients, the path to an EDS diagnosis is long and frustrating. The condition is invisible on standard imaging. X-rays show no bone damage. MRIs reveal no obvious pathology. Blood tests come back normal. And because the most common subtype, hypermobile EDS (hEDS), lacks a confirmed genetic marker, there's no definitive test to confirm its presence.[6]

Other EDS subtypes, such as vascular and classical, have been identified with genetic mutations, making them easier to diagnose through genetic testing. But hEDS, the most common form, remains a clinical diagnosis based on symptoms, along with the Beighton score, a screening test often used in diagnosis.

Diagnosis relies on clinical criteria, but many doctors aren't trained to recognize these signs, especially when they present subtly or in combination with other conditions. Patients often spend years being told their pain is psychosomatic, that they're anxious, that they need to exercise more, lose weight, or manage their stress. They're sent to physical therapists who don't understand hypermobility and prescribe aggressive stretching, which worsens joint instability. They're given antidepressants and sent on their way. They're told they're too young to have this much pain. Other times, they are told their symptoms are too vague or that nothing is really wrong because the test results are normal.

This dismissal has real consequences. It delays treatment, allowing maladaptive patterns to deepen. It isolates patients, making them question their own perceptions. And it reinforces the very anxiety and hypervigilance that worsen nervous system sensitization. When you're told repeatedly that your pain isn't real, your nervous system doesn't calm down. It ramps up. The brain interprets the lack of external validation as evidence that it needs to work harder, be more vigilant, and guard more intently.

Research on patient experience in EDS consistently highlights this pattern of diagnostic delay and invalidation.[7] Patients report feeling gaslit by medical professionals, dismissed as hypochondriacs or attention-seekers. Many describe a sense of relief when they finally receive a diagnosis, not because it changes their symptoms, but because it validates their lived experience. The pain was real. The instability was real. The exhaustion was real. And now, finally, there's a name for it. In recent years, the push toward more standardized criteria in healthcare has actually helped the condition gain recognition. Standardization has made it easier for more patients to be diagnosed accurately by giving clinicians consistent guidelines and clearer patterns to look for. But even with this, hEDS tends to be the "invisible" subtype within EDS, contributing to diagnostic delays and skepticism from medical providers who aren't trained to recognize its signs.

Even with a diagnosis, many patients face ongoing skepticism, as EDS is poorly understood in the broader medical community. Some doctors question whether it's a "real" condition or just a catch-all label for hypermobility and chronic pain. Others acknowledge the diagnosis but dismiss its severity, treating it as a benign quirk rather than a debilitating syndrome. Patients learn to advocate for themselves. Most begin bringing research to appointments, and learn to fight for accommodations and treatments that might help. And that fight, that constant need to prove, explain, and justify, adds another layer of stress to an already overburdened nervous system.

Secondary Complications: The Dual Tax of Physical and Mental Instability

EDS rarely exists in isolation. Because connective tissue is everywhere, structural instability creates ripple effects across multiple systems. The autonomic nervous system, which regulates unconscious functions such as heart rate, blood pressure, digestion, and temperature, often becomes dysregulated.[8] Many

EDS patients develop dysautonomia, a broad category that includes conditions like Postural Orthostatic Tachycardia Syndrome (POTS). They may describe dizziness or fainting when standing, or even heart palpitations at rest. They also have difficulty regulating body temperature or gastrointestinal symptoms that seem unrelated to diet or digestion.

This reflects a nervous system stuck in imbalance, unable to switch easily between sympathetic (fight-or-flight) and parasympathetic (rest-and-digest) states. From the neuroplasticity perspective, the body "learns" this imbalance. The nervous system, already primed by structural instability, begins to default to maladaptive regulation. It overreacts to postural changes. It treats something as simple as standing as a threat, and keeps the body in a state of low-level alarm even during rest.

The cognitive and emotional toll compounds this physical dysregulation. Living with unpredictability taxes mental resources in ways that are difficult to quantify but impossible to ignore. Patients describe constant anxiety, not as a separate mental health condition, but as a direct response to the body's unreliability. Hypervigilance becomes a survival strategy, leaving them scanning for signs of instability and constantly anticipating pain. As a consequence, they regularly plan exits and accommodations for every activity. This constant state of alertness becomes ingrained in the nervous system.[9] The brain becomes wired for vigilance, treating instability as a constant threat. Cognitive resources that could be devoted to focus, memory, or creativity are instead used to manage physical vulnerability.

Research on cognitive load in EDS patients shows measurable impacts on attention, processing speed, and executive function.[10] This isn't brain damage or neurodegeneration. It's the toll of chronic vigilance. The nervous system is running too many programs at once: stabilizing joints, managing pain, monitoring for threats, and regulating automatic functions. Something has to give, and often it's the cognitive bandwidth needed for daily tasks.

Chronic fatigue is another hallmark, and it's not just the result of poor sleep or deconditioning. The energy cost of constant stabilization and guarding leaves patients depleted. Even simple activities, such as a short walk, a grocery run, or a conversation with a friend, can quickly drain reserves.[11] Over time, the nervous system associates even minor effort with exhaustion. This is another form of maladaptive learning, as the body anticipates depletion before activity even begins, reinforcing the fatigue loop. Patients describe feeling tired before they start, knowing that the effort required to stabilize their bodies through any task will exceed what most people can imagine.

Think back to the bicep curl analogy at the beginning of the chapter. If you're holding tension in dozens of muscles simultaneously, all day, every day, the fatigue isn't mysterious. It's inevitable. The body is burning through energy reserves just to maintain basic posture and movement. There's nothing left over for daily activities. And when people suggest exercise as a solution, patients often feel dismissed. They're already exercising. Constantly. Involuntarily. Their muscles are working harder than most people's do during a workout, and they never get a break.

Frequent injuries, microtears, or dislocations reinforce pain cycles. These events feed into central sensitization.[12] The nervous system that's already primed by instability becomes increasingly efficient at generating pain responses. Minor traumas can create lasting impressions in cortical maps, teaching the brain to anticipate pain even in the absence of tissue damage. A joint that has once been dislocated may hurt for weeks afterward. This isn't because the tissue hasn't healed, but because the nervous system has learned to aggressively guard that area. The brain treats the joint as perpetually vulnerable, sending pain signals as a preemptive warning.

Reflection prompt

Have you noticed how uncertainty or instability in your body shapes your mood and energy? How much of your fatigue comes not from activity itself, but from guarding against what might happen?

Overlap with Fibromyalgia: When Two Storms Converge

Some patients carry both diagnoses of fibromyalgia and EDS. On paper, these may seem contradictory. One is hypersensitivity, the other is instability. One is about the nervous system amplifying every signal. The other is about connective tissue failing to hold the body together. But in reality, they layer on top of each other, creating a more complex and debilitating picture than either condition alone.

Instability forces the nervous system into constant guarding. Hypersensitivity magnifies every signal.

Together, they create a storm where pain feels both amplified and unpredictable.[13] A patient with both may feel as though their body is both collapsing and overreacting at the same time. Imagine trying to build stability on a cracked foundation while the alarm system keeps blaring at every movement. The structural weakness demands constant compensation, but the hypersensitivity makes every compensatory movement feel like a threat.

Consider what this looks like in daily life. A patient with EDS alone might dislocate a shoulder and experience localized pain, then work to stabilize the joint and move forward. A patient with fibromyalgia alone might experience widespread amplified pain but have structurally stable joints. But a patient with both experiences the dislocation *and* the amplified pain response. The injury triggers not just local pain, but a systemic flare. The nervous system, already primed for hypersensitivity, interprets the structural failure as a catastrophic threat. Pain spreads beyond the injured joint. Fatigue intensifies. Cognitive function deteriorates. The body enters a state of heightened alarm that can last for days or weeks.

Let me give you an example based on a client's experience. Say you live with both diagnoses. You may have lived with hypermobility your whole life, but didn't get the EDS diagnosis until your thirties. By then, widespread pain had already taken hold. If you sublux your wrist reaching for a coffee mug, the local pain is expected. What isn't expected is the full-body flare that follows. Your neck locks up. Your hips ache. You can't sleep. Brain fog settles in so thick you can't remember conversations from an hour earlier. The wrist heals in a week. The systemic response takes a month to calm down.

These aren't two separate problems. It's one nervous system trying to manage both structural collapse and signal amplification simultaneously. The wrist subluxation triggered central sensitization. The central sensitization amplified the protective guarding around the wrist. The guarding spread to surrounding areas, creating compensatory tension that fed back into the pain loop. And the longer it goes on, the more entrenched the pattern becomes.

From a neuroplasticity perspective, this overlap represents two maladaptive learning processes converging. One in which the nervous system is hypersensitive to input, and another in which it is overcorrecting for structural weakness. The result is a more deeply ingrained pattern that requires addressing both the amplification (as in fibro) and the stability deficit (as in EDS). Treatment for such people often requires a careful balance. Strategies that stabilize joints without overwhelming a system already primed for hypersensitivity. Pacing becomes even more critical, and interventions like gentle movement, breathwork, and restorative sleep carry double weight.

These people often feel misunderstood, even within patient communities. They don't fit neatly into the EDS narrative because their pain doesn't always correlate with joint instability. They don't fit neatly into the fibromyalgia narrative because their symptoms include clear structural issues. They exist in the overlap, and that overlap is more common than many doctors realize. Studies suggest significant comorbidity between EDS and fibromyalgia, with some estimates placing the overlap as high as 40 to 80 percent in hypermobile patients.[14]

This isn't a coincidence. It's evidence of shared mechanisms. Both conditions involve nervous system dysregulation. Both involve maladaptive neuroplasticity. Both create feedback loops where the body's protective responses become part of the problem. The difference is the entry point. EDS enters through a structural weakness. Fibromyalgia enters through amplification. But once the nervous system begins to malfunction, the pathways converge.

Interventions and Hope: Retraining Stability

Treatment for EDS focuses less on eliminating pain outright and more on building stability. That shift in framing is important. Many patients come into treatment expecting a cure, a fix, a solution that will restore their bodies to some imagined baseline of normalcy. But EDS doesn't work that way. The connective tissue will not suddenly strengthen. The ligaments will not tighten. The goal isn't to reverse the condition. The goal is to teach the nervous system and musculoskeletal system to work together more effectively, creating functional stability where structural stability is lacking.

Muscles become the new ligaments, trained to provide the support that connective tissue cannot.[15] This isn't about building bulk or achieving aesthetic fitness. It's about training muscles to fire in the correct sequence and at the right intensity to stabilize joints during movement. Stability training often begins with simple, controlled exercises: isometric holds, resistance-band work, and chair squats. These movements strengthen without risking joints. The emphasis is on control, not intensity. Slow, deliberate movements that teach the nervous system to trust the body's capacity to stabilize itself.

Let me show you what this looks like in practice. You may have had your third shoulder dislocation in 6 months. You've been told to "strengthen your rotator cuff," so you started lifting weights. Every session leaves you in more pain.

But what if you didn't start with weights? What if you began with isometric holds at chest level? Five seconds. Then ten. Then fifteen. No movement, just tension. Your nervous system needs to learn that your shoulder can hold a load without catastrophe. After two weeks, you add slow, controlled movements through a limited range. After a month, resistance bands. After three months, light dumbbells. Six months in, you can lift overhead again. Not because your ligaments have magically tightened, but because your nervous system has learned to coordinate your muscles in a way that provides stability that your connective tissue couldn't.

Balance and proprioception drills add another layer, retraining the nervous system to sense the body's position more accurately.[16] Like recalibrating a faulty

GPS. Single-leg stands, balance board exercises, and slow weight shifts. These drills may seem simple, even trivial, but they directly address the proprioceptive deficits that contribute to instability and guarding. Over time, the brain begins to receive more reliable feedback. The internal map becomes clearer. Movements feel less uncertain. Confidence builds.

Mindful pacing is equally important, and this is where many patients struggle. Pacing isn't self-care. It's survival. It's learning to respect thresholds because ignoring them means days or weeks of consequences. For someone with EDS, pushing through a flare doesn't build resilience. It reinforces the nervous system's perception that activity is dangerous. It deepens the guarding patterns. It worsens the fatigue loop. Pacing means finding the sustainable middle ground between doing nothing and doing too much. It means breaking tasks into smaller increments. It means resting before exhaustion forces rest. It means tracking patterns to identify what activities are manageable and which ones consistently trigger flares.

Activity journals or simple pacing tools like timers can help regulate effort, preventing the push-crash cycle that worsens instability. Some patients use heart rate monitors or fitness trackers to identify when they're approaching their limits. Others rely on subjective measures: rating their energy on a scale of one to ten, noting how different activities affect their symptoms, and learning to recognize early warning signs of overexertion. The tools matter less than the practice. What matters is building awareness and acting on that awareness before the body forces you to stop.

Manual therapy also has a role, but with caution. The goal isn't to strip away all tension. Some tension is protective. The aim is to release only what's overactive while supporting stability in weaker areas. Too much release without stability training can backfire, increasing vulnerability. A skilled therapist understands this balance. They work to reduce excessive guarding in muscles that are compensating unnecessarily, while reinforcing strength and coordination in muscles that need to stabilize hypermobile joints. But this requires a therapist trained in hypermobility, which is not always easy to find. Many well-meaning therapists apply standard techniques such as aggressive stretching, deep tissue work, and high-intensity exercises that worsen instability in EDS patients.

Other patients find water-based therapy helpful, as buoyancy reduces joint stress while allowing safe strengthening.[17] Aquatic therapy provides resistance without impact, making it ideal for patients whose joints cannot tolerate traditional weight-bearing exercises. The water supports the body, reducing the need for constant muscular stabilization, which allows patients to move more freely and build strength without triggering flares. Swimming, water walking, or guided aquatic exercises can improve cardiovascular fitness, muscle endurance, and proprioception in a relatively safe environment.

These strategies aren't fully detailed here because Section Three will provide the deeper dive into implementation. But they are worth mentioning as examples of how the nervous system can be retrained through consistent, safe input. The key is consistency. Small, regular efforts compound over time. The nervous system learns through repetition. One yoga class won't fix proprioception. But yoga twice a week for six months might. One session of isometric holds won't stabilize a shoulder. But daily practice for three months might. Progress is slow, and setbacks are inevitable, but the direction matters more than the pace.

Reflection prompt

What small stability-building practice could you start today, even for five minutes? How could you make it repeatable enough that your nervous system begins to trust it?

What EDS Teaches Us About Chronic Pain

Ehlers-Danlos Syndrome challenges the simplistic narrative that chronic pain is always about tissue damage or inflammation. In EDS, the tissue is faulty, yes. The connective tissue is structurally weak. But the pain doesn't map neatly onto that weakness. Patients experience pain in joints that haven't dislocated. They experience pain long after an injury has healed. They experience widespread pain with no clear anatomical origin. This is because the pain isn't just about the connective tissue. It's about what the nervous system has learned in response to instability.

EDS illustrates, perhaps more clearly than any other condition, the role of maladaptive neuroplasticity in chronic pain. The nervous system is not passive. It doesn't just transmit signals from damaged tissue to the brain. It interprets, modulates, and sometimes generates those signals based on learned patterns. In

EDS, the nervous system knows that the body is unreliable. It learns to guard constantly, to interpret ambiguous signals as threats, to maintain a baseline state of heightened vigilance. And once those patterns are established, they persist even when the original triggers are managed.

This is why structural interventions alone, things like bracing or surgical stabilization, often don't eliminate pain in EDS patients. Stabilizing a joint surgically might reduce the frequency of dislocations, but if the nervous system has already learned to guard that area aggressively, the pain may persist. The cortical map has been rewritten. The brain expects pain in that joint. And until that expectation is addressed, through retraining and nervous system modulation, the pain will continue.

This doesn't mean EDS pain is "in the head" or psychological. It means the pain has become neurological in nature. The nervous system itself is the site of dysfunction, not because of structural brain damage, but because of learned patterns that no longer serve the body. And those patterns can be unlearned, slowly and imperfectly, through the kinds of interventions described above.

Setting the Stage for What's Next

Fibromyalgia shows what happens when the nervous system over-amplifies. Ehlers–Danlos shows what happens when structure collapses. Both funnel into the same nervous system story: maladaptive plasticity reinforcing pain patterns. But what happens when the trigger isn't diffuse hypersensitivity or structural collapse, but a single injury that refuses to resolve? That's where CRPS takes the stage.

In the next chapter, we'll see how Complex Regional Pain Syndrome represents yet another doorway into the same cycle, not from instability or systemic amplification alone, but from a single injury that spirals into hypersensitivity across the entire system. CRPS is what happens when a single spark ignites a wildfire, spreading pain far beyond its source. It's the nervous system's most dramatic failure, revealing just how far the body can spiral when protective mechanisms misfire.

Endnotes

[1] Ibrahim, M. M., Shelbourne, K. D., & Freeman, J. W. (2012). *Proprioception deficits in patients with joint hypermobility syndrome.* Clinical Orthopaedics and Related Research, 470(10), 2889–2897.

[2] Dupuy, E. G., Leconte, P., Vlamynck, E., Sultan, A., Chesneau, C., Denise, P., ... & Decker, L. M. (2017). Ehlers-Danlos Syndrome, Hypermobility Type: Impact of Somatosensory Orthoses on Postural Control (A Pilot Study). *Frontiers in Human Neuroscience*, 11, 283.

[3] Hansen, N., Kass-Iliyya, L., Namer, B., Saffer, D., Lampert, A., & Faber, C. G. (2019). Central sensitization in Ehlers-Danlos syndromes: An overlooked complication with consequences. *European Journal of Pain*, 23(7), 1199-1206.

[4] Scheper, M. C., Rombaut, L., de Vries, J. E., De Wandele, I., van der Esch, M., Visser, B., ... & Engelbert, R. H. (2017). The association between muscle strength and activity limitations in patients with the hypermobility type of Ehlers-Danlos syndrome: The impact of proprioception. *Disability and Rehabilitation*, 39(14), 1391-1397.

[5] Scheper, M. C., Nicholson, L. L., & Engelbert, R. H. (2017). *Chronic pain in hypermobility syndrome and

Ehlers–Danlos syndrome—Hypermobility type: it is a challenge. Journal of Pain Research, 10, 1169–1178.

[6] Malfait, F., Francomano, C., Byers, P., Belmont, J., Berglund, B., Black, J., ... & Tinkle, B. (2017). The 2017 international classification of the Ehlers-Danlos syndromes. *American Journal of Medical Genetics Part C: Seminars in Medical Genetics*, 175(1), 8-26.

[7] Anderson, L. K., & Lane, K. R. (2021). The diagnostic journey in adults with hypermobile Ehlers-Danlos syndrome and hypermobility spectrum disorders. *Journal of the American Association of Nurse Practitioners*, 34(4), 639-648.

[8] De Wandele, I., Rombaut, L., Leybaert, L., Van de Borne, P., De Backer, T., Malfait, F., ... & Calders, P. (2014). Dysautonomia and its underlying mechanisms in the hypermobility type of Ehlers-Danlos syndrome. *Seminars in Arthritis and Rheumatism*, 44(1), 93-100.

[9] Baeza-Velasco, C., Gély-Nargeot, M. C., & Bulbena, A. (2018). *Joint hypermobility, anxiety, and psychosomatic symptoms: The link and the role of autonomic hyperarousal.* Journal of Psychosomatic Research, 111, 77–82.

[10] Glans, M., Humble, M. B., Elwin, M., & Bejerot, S. (2024). Neuropsychological Function and the

Relationship Between Subjective Cognition, Objective Cognition, and Symptoms in Hypermobile Ehlers-Danlos Syndrome. *APMR Reports*, 4(3), 100045.

[11] Castori, M., Morlino, S., Celletti, C., Ghibellini, G., Bruschini, M., Grammatico, P., ... & Camerota, F. (2013). Re-writing the natural history of pain and related symptoms in the joint hypermobility syndrome/Ehlers-Danlos syndrome, hypermobility type. *American Journal of Medical Genetics Part A*, 161(12), 2989-3004.

[12] Woolf, C. J. (2011). Central sensitization: Implications for the diagnosis and treatment of pain. *Pain*, 152(3 Suppl), S2-S15.

[13] Fairweather, D., Bruno, K. A., Darakjian, A. A., Bruce, B. K., Gehin, J. M., Kotha, A., Jain, A., Peng, Z., Hodge, D. O., Rozen, T. D., Munipalli, B., Rivera, F. A., Malavet, P. A., & Knight, D. R. T. (2023). High overlap in patients diagnosed with hypermobile Ehlers-Danlos syndrome or hypermobile spectrum disorders with fibromyalgia and 40 self-reported symptoms and comorbidities. Frontiers in Medicine, 10, 1096180.

[14] Fairweather, D., Bruno, K. A., Darakjian, A. A., Bruce, B. K., Gehin, J. M., Kotha, A., ... & Knight, D. R. T. (2023). High overlap in patients diagnosed with hypermobile

Ehlers-Danlos syndrome or hypermobility spectrum disorders with fibromyalgia and 40 self-reported symptoms and comorbidities. *Frontiers in Medicine*, 10, 1096180.

[15] Palmer, S., Bailey, S., Barker, L., Barney, L., & Elliott, A. (2014). The effectiveness of therapeutic exercise for joint hypermobility syndrome: A systematic review. *Physiotherapy*, 100(3), 220-227.

[16] Ferrell, W. R., Tennant, N., Sturrock, R. D., Ashton, L., Creed, G., Brydson, G., & Rafferty, D. (2004). Amelioration of symptoms by enhancement of proprioception in patients with joint hypermobility syndrome. *Arthritis & Rheumatism*, 50(10), 3323-3328.

[17] Bathen, T., Hångmann, A. B., Hoff, M., Andersen, L. Ø., & Rand-Hendriksen, S. (2013). Multidisciplinary treatment of disability in Ehlers-Danlos syndrome hypermobility type/hypermobility syndrome: A pilot study using a combination of physical and cognitive-behavioral therapy on 12 women. *American Journal of Medical Genetics Part A*, 161(12), 3005-3011.

Chapter Six

Other Conditions That Hijack the Pain System

A broken wrist. A tick bite. A car accident. A bout of COVID. Different triggers, different timelines, different diagnoses. But walk into any chronic pain support group, and you'll hear the same complaints: burning pain that spreads, brain fog that won't lift, fatigue that crashes you after minor effort, a body that feels like it's betraying you.

What's happening?

In the last chapters, we looked at fibromyalgia and Ehlers–Danlos. Fibro showed us what happens when the nervous system runs into overdrive, amplifying signals from the inside out. EDS showed us what happens when the body's connective tissue collapses, sending confusing input from the outside in. Both enter through different doorways. Both end in the same place: altered maps, chronic pain loops, and a body that feels unreliable.

This chapter follows that same pattern across a broader range of conditions. Whether it begins with trauma, infection, or autonomic dysfunction, the result is the same. The pain system gets hijacked by maladaptive neuroplasticity.

Complex Regional Pain Syndrome (CRPS)

CRPS often begins after a seemingly minor injury or surgery. A broken wrist. A sprained ankle. Sometimes, it's just a small procedure. Instead of resolving normally, the pain spreads and intensifies. Patients describe burning pain, swelling, stiffness, skin color or temperature changes, and hypersensitivity that makes even light touch unbearable.[1]

Here's what patients actually report: "My hand feels like it's on fire, but when I look at it, nothing's wrong." Or, "It feels swollen, huge, like it doesn't belong to me anymore." The limb might change color, turn cold or hot to the touch, and react violently to the slightest pressure. A breeze across the skin can feel like sandpaper. Wearing a shirt with sleeves becomes impossible.

What's driving this? CRPS takes the mechanisms we've been describing, like peripheral sensitization, spinal wind-up, and cortical remapping, and amplifies them to an extreme. A minor injury triggers an alarm that never shuts off.[2] The nervous system interprets every sensation in that limb as a threat. Inflammatory chemicals flood the injury site. Local nerves get sensitized, firing at lower and lower thresholds.[3]

But the real chaos happens centrally. The spinal cord and brain ramp up danger processing. As we saw in Chapter Two, central sensitization occurs when the nervous system becomes hypersensitive, amplifying normal or mild sensations into painful ones. In CRPS, this amplification is pushed to the extreme. The sensory map of the affected limb starts to blur. The brain loses crisp boundaries of where the limb begins and ends.[4]

This is cortical smudging in action. The brain's representation of the hand or foot becomes blurred and, at times, fragmented. Patients aren't imagining the "wrongness" they feel. Their brain's map no longer matches reality. Research shows that the more extensive this cortical reorganization, the more severe the pain tends to be.[5] On top of that, the sympathetic nervous system (fight-or-flight wiring) becomes abnormally linked to pain pathways.[6] Stress flares symptoms. Anxiety makes it worse. The result is a vicious loop in which small inputs, such as movement, touch, or temperature changes, trigger outsized pain and autonomic reactions.

You've been told it's all in your head. That the pain can't be that bad, that maybe you're depressing yourself into disability. But CRPS is real. The nervous system is misfiring, the brain is stuck in a loop, and no amount of positive thinking will flip the switch. The first step toward healing is believing that what you feel is legitimate, because it is.

The Role of Nerve Sprouting

As we discussed in Chapter Four, nerve sprouting after injury can add fuel to the fire. When nerves are damaged, they try to regrow. When nerves sprout new branches, the goal is to restore communication. Sometimes it works. Other times, especially in conditions like CRPS, the growth becomes disorganized. Instead of improving signaling, the overlapping branches introduce additional noise and hypersensitivity into an already sensitized system. The brain receives this noisy, confusing input and interprets it as danger. This magnifies the threat response, reinforces the cortical smudging, and deepens the sensitization.

Remember our analogy about tuning in to a radio station? When you're on the right frequency, the signal is clear. But move one notch off, and you start picking up fragments of the station mixed with static and interference from adjacent channels. The music is still there, but it's buried in noise. That's what nerve sprouting creates in CRPS: overlapping signals that the brain struggles to parse.

The sprouting doesn't happen in isolation. It feeds directly into the cortical map alterations we just discussed. Noisy peripheral input reaches an already amplified central system. The brain tries to organize the chaos, only to amplify it further. Together, these processes create a feedback loop where structural changes at the nerve level and functional changes in the brain reinforce each other, compounding the problem with each cycle.

This is why certain interventions work so well for CRPS. Graded motor imagery, mirror therapy, desensitization exercises, and careful movement exposure all help counter the noisy signals.[7] They feed the brain cleaner information. They help redraw the map. Recovery is about retraining the system, not fixing the tissue.

Let me give you an example. Let's say someone breaks their wrist in a minor fall. The bone heals in six weeks, but the pain doesn't go away. It spreads up the arm, and the hand turns blotchy, sometimes red, sometimes pale. Anything touching the skin feels like fire. You can't wear long sleeves or even shake hands. The pain is so consuming that you stop using the arm entirely, which only makes things worse.

Starting mirror therapy might feel absurd. Watching your good hand move in a mirror while your painful hand stays still shouldn't do anything, right? But after two weeks of daily practice, something shifts. The brain, seeing the reflected hand move without pain, begins to update its map. The burning eases slightly. After a month, you can tolerate a light touch. After three months, you are using your hand again, cautiously but functionally. The tissue hadn't changed. The nerves hadn't magically healed. But the brain's interpretation of those signals had been retrained.

That's the power of understanding CRPS through the lens of neuroplasticity. The condition isn't about permanent damage. It's about a system that learned the wrong pattern and needs new information to unlearn it.

Viewed through maladaptive neuroplasticity, CRPS is trauma plus learning. An injury starts the alarm. Repeated danger signals teach the system to expect a threat in that limb. Over time, cortical remapping, spinal sensitization, and limbic amplification (fear, frustration, vigilance) reinforce each other. The system learns too well and forgets how to reset.

Reflection prompt

If you've ever felt your pain was out of proportion to the injury, or that your body part didn't feel like it belonged, you've experienced a glimpse of how CRPS reshapes maps in the brain.

Chronic Infections and Immune Overload

Picture this. You get sick. It could be a tick bite that goes unnoticed for weeks. It could be COVID or even prolonged exposure to mold in a building. The acute phase passes, but you never quite bounce back. Fatigue drags on, brain fog settles in, and pain spreads through your body with no clear pattern. Small efforts, like walking to the mailbox or standing in the shower, leave you wrecked for days.

Welcome to the world of chronic infection and immune overload.

Whether it's Lyme disease, Long COVID, or prolonged mold exposure, the pattern is the same: an immune challenge that never fully resolves. The immune system continues to signal danger, flooding the nervous system with inflammatory mediators. The brain interprets this as a chronic threat. The system learns that exertion equals crash, and avoidance increases.[8]

From a maladaptive neuroplasticity perspective, prolonged immune signaling acts like a metronome for threat learning. It keeps time. It keeps the system alert. It keeps the alarm ringing at a low, constant hum. Microglia, the brain's immune cells, become primed. Once primed, they overreact to subsequent stressors.[9] A bad night's sleep, a stressful conversation, or a bit of physical exertion can trigger an exaggerated inflammatory response in the brain. This isn't psychosomatic. It's neuroimmune.

Interoceptive signals (heartbeat, breathing, gut sensations) get interpreted through a threat-biased lens. The brain scans internal sensations for danger and finds it everywhere. Fatigue deepens. Pain spreads. Autonomic dysregulation kicks in, leading to orthostatic intolerance, thermoregulatory intolerance, and sleep disruption.[10] Thresholds drop. The nervous system pairs exertion with collapse. The loop conditions itself.

Viral infections, including COVID, don't just activate the immune system. They activate old neural pathways associated with prior illness, injury, or threat. The nervous system remembers those patterns, and once the immune system is under stress, those pathways can re-ignite. This is one reason long COVID can feel strangely familiar to people who previously had EBV (Epstein-Barr) related illness or chronic pain. The body isn't reliving the past; the nervous system is reactivating a pattern it learned a long time ago.

Regarding chronic Lyme disease, debates about it have turned patients into victims of medical politics. Some doctors believe in it, while others do not. As the argument continues, you may find yourself questioning whether your own decline is real. You're not. Whether the infection is still active or your immune system is still responding, the symptoms are real and deserve to be addressed. You don't need permission to feel what you feel.

Brain Fog and the Cognitive Toll

One of the most disabling aspects of these conditions is cognitive dysfunction. Brain fog is more than forgetting where you put your keys. It's neural networks overwhelmed by inflammatory signaling, leaving less capacity for attention, working memory, and processing speed.[11] Words disappear mid-sentence. Thoughts scatter. Simple tasks feel insurmountable.

This mirrors fibro fog but stems from a different trigger. In fibromyalgia, the amplification comes from within. Here, it starts with an external invader (a virus, bacteria, or toxin) that leaves a lasting imprint on the immune system and the brain. The chronic activation doesn't just affect pain pathways. It taxes every cognitive system, making it harder to think clearly, remember details, or maintain focus for more than a few minutes.

Patients describe it as trying to think through a thick cloud. You reach for a word, and it's gone. You start a task and forget why you started it. You read the same paragraph three times and still can't retain the information. This isn't laziness or lack of effort. It's a brain running too many background processes, with inflammation consuming resources that would otherwise be available for clear thinking. You're not doing anything wrong. The system is just overloaded. That's what chronic immune activation does to cognitive function. It hijacks resources, leaving less bandwidth for everything else.

The work of recovery involves carefully titrated activity, symptom-paced exposures, sleep support, and nervous-system-calming inputs. The goal isn't to push through. It's to help the brain relearn safety without provoking collapse. Small, consistent inputs. Gradual exposure. Patience with setbacks. The system can unlearn the crash response, but it takes time.

What makes this particularly frustrating is the variability. Some days you might feel almost clear. Other days, the fog descends without warning, and even simple decisions feel impossible. This unpredictability makes it hard to plan, hard to commit to activities, and hard to explain to others why you're struggling. But the variability itself is part of the pattern. The immune system's reactivity fluctuates based on sleep, stress, activity level, and a dozen other factors. Understanding this doesn't make it easier, but it does make it less mysterious.

This may describe it perfectly: You used to be able to manage three things at once. Now you can barely manage one. And some days, even that one thing feels like climbing a mountain. That's the reality of living with chronic immune activation. Every cognitive task requires more effort than it should, and the effort itself can trigger a crash.

Reflection prompt

Have you noticed how even small efforts can lead to a disproportionate crash? That's your nervous system pairing exertion with danger. And it can be unlearned with the right pacing and inputs.

PTSD and Trauma-Linked Pain

Not all wounds are visible. Traumatic experiences can change the body's wiring, teaching the nervous system to remain alert long after the threat has passed. These experiences leave more than emotional scars; trauma manifests physically in the body.

In Chapter Three, we explored how trauma rewires the limbic system, keeping it in a state of high alert. In PTSD and related trauma-linked pain states, this rewiring doesn't just amplify emotional reactivity. It also embeds itself in the body. Pain becomes part of the trauma signature. Muscles brace in patterns learned during the original threat. Sensations that should feel neutral get flagged as dangerous. The body remembers what the mind tries to forget.[12]

Triggers don't need to be dramatic. Context, memory, or subtle cues can reactivate the alarm. A smell. A sound. A particular time of day. Fear learning strengthens salience networks (what the brain pays attention to) and weakens inhibitory control.[13] Normal sensations get scanned for danger and amplified. A tight muscle becomes a warning. A flutter in the chest becomes a crisis. Avoidance reduces corrective experiences, which prevents the system from relearning safety.

Think of it like an alarm system that becomes too sensitive. It sounds off for every gust of wind, every passing car, every shadow. Because it's always going off, the system never learns what true safety feels like. The alarm becomes the baseline.

Trauma doesn't just live in your mind. It lives in your body; in the tightness of your shoulders, the ache in your chest, the pain that shows up in places that make no anatomical sense. You've been told to "let it go," to "move on," to "think positive." But healing trauma isn't about thinking differently. It's about teaching your nervous system that the threat is over, and that takes time, patience, and safety.

Trauma Reshapes the Map

Trauma doesn't just activate the limbic system. It can also reshape cortical maps by reinforcing hypervigilance to certain sensations.[14] This creates the same kind of blurring seen in CRPS, but driven by memory and context rather than physical injury. The brain over-represents threat-associated areas of the body. Muscles that were tense during the trauma stay tense. Pain patterns that emerged during the event become ingrained. The map gets redrawn around danger, not function.

Consider what this looks like in practice. Someone experiences a car accident. At the moment of impact, their neck whips forward, their shoulders brace, their jaw clenches. The accident is brief, but the body remembers. Weeks later, the tissue has healed, but the neck still feels tight. The shoulders still carry tension. The jaw still aches. Not because the injury persists, but because the nervous system learned to hold that pattern during a moment of extreme threat. And now, even without conscious awareness, the body maintains that defensive posture.

This is why trauma-linked pain often doesn't respond to standard treatments. You can massage the tight muscles, but they tighten right back up. You can stretch the neck, but the stiffness returns. The problem isn't in the tissue. It's in the map. The brain has associated that area of the body with danger, and until that association is addressed, the pattern will persist. Gradual, supported exposure (to movement, to sensation, to contexts that used to provoke flares) alongside regulation skills (breath, grounding, cognitive reframing) provides new learning that loosens the bond between pain and fear.[15] This isn't about forcing someone to "just relax." It's about giving the nervous system safe experiences that contradict the old pattern. Over time, those new experiences accumulate. The map can shift. The alarm can quiet.

It's important to understand that this process doesn't invalidate the trauma. It doesn't minimize what happened. What it does is recognize that the body's protective response, while adaptive in the moment, has outlived its usefulness. The threat is gone, but the protection remains. And that protection, held for too long, becomes the problem.

POTS and Dysautonomia

Stand up. Your heart races. Vision tunnels. The world tilts. You grab the counter to keep from collapsing. This isn't anxiety. This is your autonomic nervous system failing to regulate blood flow and heart rate.

Welcome to POTS (Postural Orthostatic Tachycardia Syndrome) and the broader world of dysautonomia. These conditions involve instability in the autonomic nervous system, the circuitry that regulates heart rate, blood pressure, digestion, temperature, and other automatic functions. Symptoms include dizziness or faintness on standing, racing heart, brain fog, fatigue, GI upset, temperature intolerance, and sleep disruption.[16] Dysautonomia commonly overlaps with hypermobility/EDS, post-infectious syndromes, and fibromyalgia.

Although not a "pain disorder" per se, dysautonomia feeds the chronic pain loop in profound ways. When the sympathetic system stays dominant and the parasympathetic system stays suppressed, the body lives in a state of constant low-grade alarm. Blood flow to the brain becomes unreliable. Reduced cerebral perfusion (less efficient blood flow to the brain on standing) worsens fog and fatigue.[17] The brain interprets this instability as danger and lowers thresholds for pain. Internal sensations (rapid heartbeat, breathlessness, dizziness) get tagged as threats. The system learns to expect instability, and over time, that expectation becomes the pattern.

You've been told you're "just anxious." That standing up shouldn't make your heart race. Maybe you need therapy, not a cardiologist. But POTS isn't anxiety. It's your autonomic nervous system failing to regulate itself, and that's measurable, real, and exhausting. You're not imagining the dizziness, the fatigue, or the brain fog. Your body is struggling to keep up with basic tasks, and that deserves to be taken seriously.

Mast cell activation syndrome (MCAS) shows up frequently in the same population that struggles with POTS, EDS, and chronic pain conditions. Mast cells are part of the immune system and release chemical mediators, such as histamine, that help the body respond to injury or infection. In MCAS, these cells become overly sensitive and release those chemicals far too easily, often in response to everyday stimuli: heat, stress, certain foods, pressure on the skin, even changes in posture. This constant, low-grade release creates a background of inflammation that can amplify pain, worsen fatigue, disrupt the gut, and heighten autonomic instability. It keeps the nervous system in a state of readiness, as if something is always "about to go wrong," reinforcing the same threat-driven loops seen in dysautonomia and chronic pain. You don't need full-blown allergic reactions to experience MCAS symptoms; for many people, it simply adds another layer of reactivity that makes everything else more challenging to manage.

The Faulty Thermostat

Think of dysautonomia like a faulty thermostat. A working thermostat keeps the temperature steady. It senses changes and adjusts automatically. A broken thermostat swings wildly between extremes. The house is freezing one minute, sweltering the next. Nothing stabilizes.

That's what happens in the autonomic nervous system with POTS. Heart rate and blood pressure swing erratically. The body never finds equilibrium. The nervous system interprets this fluctuation as a threat, which reinforces sensitization and feeds into the chronic pain loop.

Supporting autonomic balance (hydration, salt, compression garments, recumbent conditioning, paced activity) helps because it reduces background noise and provides the nervous system with a steadier signal to learn from.[18] These interventions don't cure dysautonomia, but they provide the system with more predictable input. When the fluctuations become less extreme, the brain has less reason to stay on high alert. The alarm tone quiets, just a bit. And that small shift can make a meaningful difference in daily function.

The brain fog that comes with POTS deserves special mention. When blood flow to the brain drops, even briefly, cognitive function takes a hit. Words disappear. Thoughts feel sluggish. Memory falters. This isn't psychological. It's mechanical. The brain isn't getting the fuel it needs.

Over time, the nervous system learns to anticipate this lack and becomes hypervigilant to internal sensations, which paradoxically worsens the symptoms. You start scanning your body constantly: Is my heart racing? Am I about to pass out? Do I need to sit down? That constant monitoring, while understandable, keeps the system on edge. The more you scan, the more you notice. The more you notice, the more the system interprets those sensations as threats. And the cycle continues.

Addressing the autonomic instability helps, but so does retraining the brain's interpretation of those signals. Learning to recognize that a racing heart doesn't always mean danger, or that dizziness doesn't always mean collapse. This cognitive shift, combined with physical interventions, can help break the loop.

You may be someone with POTS who can't stand for more than five minutes without feeling faint. You've been told it was anxiety, possibly even been given antidepressants. Three different doctors have dismissed you before finally getting a diagnosis. Once you understand what was happening, that your blood wasn't pooling properly when you stood, that your heart was racing to compensate, that your brain wasn't getting enough oxygen, you can start addressing it.

You can increase your salt and fluid intake. You start wearing compression stockings. You do recumbent exercises that don't trigger your symptoms. And slowly, your tolerance improves. Not because the underlying condition disappeared, but because you gave your nervous system the support it needs to function better. Six months later, you can stand for twenty minutes. A year later, you can walk through a grocery store without collapsing. The progress is slow, but it is real. Progress with POTS isn't always this perfectly linear. There are good weeks and bad ones, but over time, the trend can move in a positive direction.

Reflection prompt

If you've ever stood up and felt the world go sideways, or noticed that your symptoms flare when your body can't regulate temperature or heart rate, you're seeing dysautonomia in action. This isn't weakness. It's wiring.

Why They Make Sense Together

On the surface, CRPS, chronic Lyme, Long COVID, mold illness, PTSD, and POTS appear very different. One begins with a minor fracture. Another with a virus. Another with a traumatic memory. Another with blood-flow instability. But beneath the surface, the pattern is consistent.

Each condition ties back to the same mechanisms we described in Section One.

Start with a trigger. Injury, infection, toxin, or trauma initiates alarm signaling. The body responds appropriately at first. Pain, inflammation, immune activation, or vigilance all serve protective functions in the short term. But then something goes wrong. The signaling doesn't shut off. Inflammatory mediators keep circulating. Autonomic imbalance persists. Limbic hypervigilance remains locked in. The system stays in "threat learning" mode.

This is where maladaptive neuroplasticity takes over. Repeated pairing of sensation and threat reconfigures the system. Spinal sensitization increases gain. Cortical maps become amplified or blurred. Salience networks (anterior insula and dorsal anterior cingulate cortex) prioritize danger. Descending inhibitory pathways (the brakes) weaken.[19] The brain starts predicting pain and threat, then perceives incoming signals through that prediction.[20] Neutral input is more likely to be labeled as danger. Real danger is magnified. The system becomes hypersensitive to everything.

Behavioral conditioning completes the loop. Avoidance and guarding reduce corrective experiences. The system doesn't get the data it needs to update the model. Rest becomes isolation. Caution becomes fear. The loop sustains itself.[21]

They look different, but they rhyme. Variations on the same maladaptive neuroplasticity theme. This is why different catalysts end in similar day-to-day realities: fatigue, brain fog, pain flares, poor recovery, and unpredictability. They are not identical conditions, but they follow the same logic of a nervous system that has learned too well and forgotten how to reset.

The practical implication is hopeful. If learning wires these patterns in, new learning can wire them out. Not instantly, and not by willpower alone, but through carefully chosen inputs repeated over time. Movement that rebuilds maps. Exposures that disconfirm threat. Sleep that restores inhibitory control. Autonomic support that quiets the noise. Cognitive and emotional practices that change interpretation. The tools are the same because the underlying problem is the same.

Closing

Fibro showed us overdrive. EDS showed us collapse. This chapter shows us how trauma, infection, and imbalance can all pull the same system off course. The details differ, but the destination is the same: chronic pain and fatigue rooted in maladaptive neuroplasticity.

These conditions are not random. They are not meaningless. They are the predictable outcomes of a system that learns too well and fails to reset. The pain is real. The suffering is real. The confusion is real. And the path forward, while not simple, follows the same logic in reverse.

You are not broken beyond repair. Your nervous system is stuck in a pattern it learned. And just as it followed the same logic into dysfunction, it can follow the same logic out, with the right tools and inputs.

Before we move on to those tools, the next chapter explains why this lens matters. How understanding pain this way validates your experience, gives you language for conversations with providers, and makes the treatments in Section Three make sense. Because once you see the pattern, you can't unsee it. And that clarity is the first step toward change.

Endnotes

[1] Birklein, F., & Schlereth, T. (2015). Complex regional pain syndrome—significant progress in understanding. *Pain*, 156(Suppl 1), S94-S103.

[2] Marinus, J., Moseley, G. L., Birklein, F., Baron, R., Maihöfner, C., Kingery, W. S., & van Hilten, J. J. (2011). Clinical features and pathophysiology of complex regional pain syndrome. Lancet Neurology, 10(7), 637-648.

[3] Uceyler, N., Eberle, T., Rolke, R., Birklein, F., & Sommer, C. (2007). Differential expression patterns of cytokines in complex regional pain syndrome. *Pain*, 132(1-2), 195-205.

[4] Maihöfner, C., et al. (2004). Cortical reorganization during recovery from complex regional pain syndrome. *Neurology*, 63(4), 693-701.

[5] Maihöfner, C., Handwerker, H. O., Neundörfer, B., & Birklein, F. (2003). Patterns of cortical reorganization in complex regional pain syndrome. *Neurology*, 61(12), 1707-1715.

[6] Harden, R. N., et al. (2013). Complex regional pain syndrome: Practical diagnostic and treatment guidelines. *Pain Medicine*, 14(2), 180-229.

[7] Bowering, K. J., et al. (2013). The effects of graded motor imagery and its components on chronic pain: A systematic review and meta-analysis. *The Journal of Pain*, 14(1), 3-13.

[8] Proal, A. D., & Marshall, T. G. (2018). Myalgic encephalomyelitis/chronic fatigue syndrome in the era of the human microbiome. *Microbiome*, 6, 120.

[9] Nakatomi, Y., et al. (2014). Neuroinflammation in patients with chronic fatigue syndrome/myalgic

encephalomyelitis. *Journal of Nuclear Medicine*, 55(6), 945-950.

[10] Barnden, L. R., Crouch, B., Kwiatek, R., Burnet, R., Del Fante, P., & MacKay, C. (2011). A brain MRI study of chronic fatigue syndrome: Evidence of brainstem dysfunction and altered autonomic regulation. *NMR in Biomedicine*, 24(10), 1302–1311.

[11] Morris, G., et al. (2016). Myalgic encephalomyelitis or chronic fatigue syndrome: How could the illness develop? *Metabolic Brain Disease*, 31(3), 385-415.

[12] van der Kolk, B. A. (2014). *The Body Keeps the Score: Brain, Mind, and Body in the Healing of Trauma*. Viking.

[13] Norrholm, S. D., et al. (2011). Fear extinction in traumatized civilians with posttraumatic stress disorder. *Biological Psychiatry*, 69(6), 556-563.

[14] Hayes, J. P., et al. (2012). Quantitative meta-analysis of neural activity in posttraumatic stress disorder. *Biology of Mood & Anxiety Disorders*, 2, 9.

[15] Foa, E. B., et al. (2007). Randomized trial of prolonged exposure for posttraumatic stress disorder with and without cognitive restructuring. *Journal of Consulting and Clinical Psychology*, 75(6), 904-913.

[16] Raj, S. R. (2013). Postural tachycardia syndrome (POTS). *Circulation*, 127(23), 2336-2342.

[17] Stewart, J. M., et al. (2012). Mechanisms of sympathetic regulation in orthostatic intolerance. *Journal of Applied Physiology*, 113(10), 1659-1668.

[18] Benarroch, E. E. (2012). Postural tachycardia syndrome: A heterogeneous and multifactorial disorder. *Mayo Clinic Proceedings*, 87(12), 1214-1225.

[19] Woolf, C. J. (2011). Central sensitization: Implications for the diagnosis and treatment of pain. *Pain*, 152(3 Suppl), S2-S15.

[20] Büchel, C., et al. (2014). Placebo analgesia: A predictive coding perspective. *Neuron*, 81(6), 1223-1239.

[21] Vlaeyen, J. W., & Linton, S. J. (2012). Fear-avoidance model of chronic musculoskeletal pain: 12 years on. *Pain*, 153(6), 1144-1147.

Chapter Seven

Why This Lens Matters

If You're Collecting Diagnoses

Let's start here. If you've been diagnosed with more than one of these conditions, you're not alone. In fact, you're the norm.

EDS and POTS. Fibromyalgia and MCAS. Chronic Lyme and PTSD. Long COVID and dysautonomia. These conditions don't travel solo. They cluster and overlap. They show up together so often that researchers and clinicians have begun using terms such as "comorbidity" and "syndrome overlap" to describe the pattern. But those terms don't capture what it actually feels like to live through it.

It feels like collecting diagnoses, like every specialist adds another label to the pile, and your medical chart becomes a list of mysteries no one can solve. It feels like bad luck, almost like your body is failing in every possible direction at once. And when you mention this pattern to doctors, some dismiss it. Others look confused, like you're an anomaly they can't categorize. A few suggest, subtly or not, that it's all in your head.

But here's what they're missing. This isn't bad luck. This is predictable.

And understanding why, understanding the pattern you've been living, is the first step toward reclaiming your life.

One Vulnerable System, Multiple Expressions

Think back to everything we've covered in Section Two. Fibromyalgia is a nervous system stuck in overdrive, amplifying signals. EDS is connective tissue that can't stabilize the body, leaving the nervous system flooded with confusing proprioceptive input. CRPS is trauma that rewires the pain map. Chronic infections prime the immune system and sensitize the brain. PTSD keeps the limbic system locked in threat mode. POTS is an autonomic instability that creates constant background noise.

Now ask yourself. Your nervous system is already sensitized (fibro), and your connective tissue is already unstable (EDS). Your immune system is already primed (post-infection), your autonomic system is already dysregulated (POTS), and you have a history of trauma (PTSD). So why wouldn't these conditions appear together?

They're not only separate diseases. They're different expressions of the same vulnerable system under various kinds of stress.[1] A sensitized nervous system doesn't just amplify pain. It also misinterprets autonomic signals (hello, POTS), overreacts to immune activity (hello, MCAS), and struggles to regulate after trauma (hello, PTSD). Unstable connective tissue doesn't just cause hypermobility. It also disrupts proprioception, which can alter cortical maps (fibro) and feed autonomic instability (POTS). Immune priming doesn't just cause fatigue. It also lowers pain thresholds, disrupts sleep, and worsens brain fog. To be clear here, I am not suggesting that if you have had any of these symptoms at some point, that you have that condition. It is way more complex than this. I am simply demonstrating what it looks like for someone who does have those conditions stacked on top of each other.

These systems talk to each other. When one fails, it destabilizes the others. And in a body that's already vulnerable, whether through genetics, trauma, infection, or injury, the dominoes fall fast.

Here's how it actually happens. Start with structural instability in EDS. Joints that move too far send noisy, contradictory proprioceptive signals to the brain. The brain's body map becomes blurred, making it harder to stabilize movement without excessive muscular guarding. That constant guarding rarely relaxes, keeping the nervous system in a state of low-grade alarm. Over time, this environment can prime central sensitization, which is why fibromyalgia so often appears alongside EDS.

The same chronic sympathetic activation that drives guarding can also destabilize the autonomic nervous system. For some people, that means POTS-type symptoms: difficulty regulating blood flow, dizziness on standing, and a heart that races to compensate. Autonomic instability then disrupts sleep, which further lowers pain thresholds and worsens cognitive function.

If there's a history of trauma, common in both EDS and fibro populations, the limbic system stays hypervigilant, interpreting every flare as proof the body isn't safe. PTSD symptoms can emerge or intensify. The immune system, strained by chronic sympathetic overdrive and poor sleep, becomes reactive. Mast cells destabilize, and MCAS comes into play.

This isn't a strict sequence but an interconnected web of feedback loops. Each system influences the others. Structural instability feeds sensory confusion, which fuels guarding and sympathetic activation, in turn disrupting autonomic balance and immune stability. These conditions don't simply coexist. They reinforce each other, creating a network of vulnerabilities that can feel impossible to untangle. But once you see the pattern, it no longer looks random. It looks like a cascade. And cascades, once recognized, can be interrupted.

Why Interventions May Have Felt Incomplete

This also explains why so many interventions feel frustrating or incomplete. Exercise, sleep hygiene, stress management, and manual therapy: these aren't wrong. But if they're applied only through the old paradigm (pain equals damage, fix the structure), they often disappoint. A person lifts weights and flares up, so they quit. A therapist releases tight muscles, but the relief doesn't last. Sleep is encouraged, but nobody explains why it matters or how to approach it when pain keeps you awake.

Through this lens, the same tools take on new meaning. Let's revisit them, not as isolated interventions, but as ways to address the underlying nervous system dysfunction that ties all these conditions together.

Movement isn't just about building strength or restoring range of motion. It's about retraining the brain's map of the body. When someone with fibromyalgia or EDS flares after exercise, it doesn't prove they're broken. It's evidence that their nervous system is interpreting new input as a threat. Research on graded motor imagery and mirror therapy demonstrates that movement-based interventions can literally reshape cortical representations of the body, reducing pain by teaching the brain that movement is safe.[2] Scaling back the dose and repeating it gradually is like teaching the body a new language. Each repetition tells the brain, *this is safe*, until the map begins to redraw itself. The goal isn't to push through pain or prove toughness. The goal is to provide the nervous system with repeated exposure to safe movement, allowing it to begin relearning what normal feels like.

Sleep isn't just rest. As we discussed in Chapter Two, it's when the nervous system resets and rewires. Poor sleep doesn't just leave you tired; it leaves your nervous system more sensitive. Studies show that sleep deprivation increases sensitivity to pain by disrupting descending inhibitory pathways and heightening activity in pain-processing regions, such as the anterior cingulate cortex.[3] Deep, restorative sleep is when inhibitory pathways strengthen, and pain signals quiet. Understanding this makes sleep hygiene less of a chore and more of an investment in rewiring. For someone juggling multiple conditions, improving sleep isn't just about feeling rested. It's about giving every system (pain processing, autonomic regulation, immune function, cognitive clarity) a chance to recalibrate.

Stress regulation isn't just coping. As we explored in Chapter Three, it's dialing down limbic overdrive. When stress dominates, the amygdala amplifies every sensation. Chronic stress dysregulates the hypothalamic-pituitary-adrenal (HPA) axis, perpetuating a state of hypervigilance that keeps the nervous system primed for threat.[4] Practices like breathing, grounding, or mindfulness aren't about being trendy; they literally reduce the alarm tone in the brain, shifting the system out of sympathetic dominance and into parasympathetic recovery. For someone with POTS, calming the autonomic system can reduce tachycardia episodes. For someone with fibromyalgia, it can lower pain amplification. For someone with PTSD, it can break the cycle of hypervigilance. Same intervention, multiple benefits, because they all share the same root dysfunction.

Manual therapy isn't just loosening tissue. It's giving the brain new input. A massage or gentle mobilization can temporarily change how the brain interprets a region of the body. The relief doesn't last if the nervous system immediately reverts to its old map. But combined with movement and awareness, it becomes part of a bigger retraining process. Research suggests that manual therapy may work in part by modulating pain through changes in cortical processing rather than purely mechanical effects on tissue.[5] This is why manual therapy alone sometimes disappoints, but manual therapy as part of a comprehensive approach (movement, sleep, nervous system regulation) can be transformative.

It's not that the tools were wrong. It's that the paradigm was incomplete. Reframing them through the lens of maladaptive neuroplasticity offers a different outcome, one that feels more coherent and more effective. When you understand that exercise isn't about "fixing" weak muscles but about teaching your nervous system to trust movement again, the approach changes. When you know that sleep isn't optional but essential for nervous system recalibration, it becomes a priority. When you understand that stress management isn't self-care fluff but a direct intervention on limbic amplification, you stop dismissing it.

These interventions work because they target the shared mechanisms beneath all these conditions. And when you address the root system, you don't just improve one condition. You improve all of them at once.

The Diagnostic Odyssey

Here's how it usually goes. You start with one thing. It could be joint pain that won't quit, fatigue after an infection, or dizziness whenever you stand. You see a doctor. They run tests. The tests come back normal, or they may show something minor: mild hypermobility, slightly elevated inflammatory markers, or a positive Lyme test. You get a diagnosis. You try treatments. Some help a little. Some don't help at all. And then something else starts.

Now it's brain fog. Now it's gut issues. Now it's temperature intolerance, exercise intolerance, or pain spreading to places that were fine before. You see more specialists. You collect more diagnoses. Each one is treated in isolation, as if it has nothing to do with the others. Your rheumatologist focuses on the EDS. Your cardiologist focuses on the POTS. Your pain management doctor focuses on the fibro. Your infectious disease doctor focuses on Lyme disease. No one is looking at the whole picture.

And you're left wondering: how did this happen? Why me? Am I just falling apart?

The answer is no. You're not falling apart. You're experiencing one system expressing dysfunction through multiple channels. The fact that these conditions cluster together isn't evidence that you're uniquely unlucky. It's evidence that they share a root cause.

Take EDS, POTS, and fibromyalgia. You've been told the EDS explained your joint pain, the POTS explained your dizziness, and the fibromyalgia explained everything else. But no one could tell you why you had all three. No one could explain why a simple grocery trip left you with a migraine, heart palpitations, and full-body pain that lasted three days. You feel like a walking collection of broken parts, each specialist handing you a new label but no real answers.

The Pattern You Can't Unsee

Three diagnoses. One cascade. Once you see it, you'll stop blaming yourself. Stop feeling like a medical mystery. And started addressing the root system instead of chasing symptoms. And once you see it, you can't unsee it. The pain that seemed random starts to make sense. The unpredictable flares start to follow patterns. The symptoms that seemed disconnected begin to fit together.

You notice that stress flares your pain. That poor sleep tanks your energy. That pushing too hard one day crashes you the next. That certain movements feel safe and others trigger alarms. That your body isn't randomly betraying you. It's responding to inputs in predictable ways.

And when you see the pattern, you can start working with it instead of against it.

You stop asking victim questions and start asking participant questions. Not "What's wrong with me?" but "What is my nervous system reacting to?" Not "How do I make this stop?" but "What inputs can I change to help my system learn something new?"

That shift, from passive victim to active participant, is everything.

That's what this lens does. It doesn't promise a cure. It offers clarity. And clarity, for someone who's been lost in the chaos of chronic illness, is powerful.

Finding Your Words

Understanding this framework also gives you something you might not have had before: words.

Words to explain to your doctor why you're not just anxious, why the pain is real even when the test results are normal, why rest doesn't fix it, and why pushing through makes it worse.

Words to explain to your family why you can't just "power through" or "think positive," why you need boundaries and accommodations, why some days are manageable, and others aren't.

Words to explain to yourself why this is happening, why it's not your fault, and why recovery is possible even when it feels impossible.

You can say: "My nervous system learned a pattern. It's stuck in a loop. The pain is real because my brain is interpreting signals as danger even when there's no tissue damage. This isn't weakness. This is neuroplasticity gone wrong. And just like it learned this pattern, it can learn a new one."

That clarity matters. It cuts through the shame, the guilt, the self-blame. It gives you a framework to work from instead of flailing in the dark.

Talking to Providers

This framework also changes the way you can talk to your doctors, therapists, or trainers. Instead of saying, "Fix my tissue" or "Make this muscle relax," you can frame the conversation around, "Help my nervous system relearn safety." That shift matters. It shifts the dialogue from chasing structural fixes to creating experiences that provide the nervous system with new input.

For example, instead of asking, "Why does this keep tightening back up?" you might say, "How can we create repeated safe movements so my body learns not to guard so much here?" This not only clarifies what you're looking for but also shows your providers that you are engaged in the process and that you want to work with them, not just receive treatment.

Here's what that might sound like in practice:

To a physical therapist: "I know my tissues aren't damaged, but my nervous system treats this movement like a threat. Can we work on graded exposure so my brain learns it's safe?"

To a doctor seemingly dismissing your symptoms: "I understand the scans look normal. But research shows that chronic pain often involves central sensitization, in which the nervous system amplifies signals even in the absence of structural damage. Can we explore treatments that address nervous system regulation?"

To a family member who doesn't understand: "It's not that I'm not trying. My nervous system is stuck in a pattern where it interprets normal sensations as threats. I'm working on retraining it, but it takes time and consistency."

Some providers will get it immediately. Others will need time to adjust their thinking. A few won't get it at all, and that's fine. You're not responsible for educating every clinician you encounter. But by framing your experience through this lens, you're giving yourself and your providers a better chance of working together effectively. You're also giving yourself permission to seek out practitioners who understand that pain isn't always about damage, and healing isn't always about fixing what's broken.

If a provider dismisses the neuroplasticity framework entirely, or insists that everything must have a structural cause, that's helpful information. It tells you they may not be the right fit for where you are now. Finding someone who gets it, whether that's a physical therapist, a pain psychologist, or a physician trained in integrative or functional approaches, can make all the difference.

Not Five Battles. One Path Forward.

This is why Section Three of this book doesn't give you separate protocols for each condition. It provides an integrated approach that targets shared mechanisms: nervous system regulation, cortical remapping, autonomic support, trauma processing, and movement retraining.

You're not fighting five separate battles. You're reclaiming one system that learned the wrong patterns. And that system, as stuck as it might feel right now, is still capable of learning something new.

The clustering isn't proof that you're broken beyond repair. It's proof that everything is connected. And when you understand the connections, you can stop chasing symptoms and start addressing the source.

Here's what that looks like in practice. When you improve sleep, you're not just addressing fatigue. You're giving your nervous system a chance to recalibrate pain thresholds, stabilize autonomic function, and restore cognitive resources. When you calm the autonomic system through breathwork or gentle movement, you're not just managing POTS; you're also calming the autonomic system. You're reducing sympathetic overdrive, which lowers pain amplification and improves emotional regulation. When you practice graded movement exposure, you're not just building strength. You're teaching your brain that movement is safe, which reduces guarding, improves proprioception, and restores confidence in your body.

Same interventions. Multiple benefits. Because the conditions aren't separate, they're facets of the same underlying dysfunction. Address the root, and the ripple effects reach everywhere.

Preparing for Change

This chapter is not about false hope. Understanding the mechanism doesn't mean the road ahead will be easy, quick, or simple. But it does mean there is a road. It means pain is not random, and healing is not impossible. It reframes the discouraging experiences of the past, the exercises that flared, the treatments that didn't last, the advice that sounded hollow, as pieces of a bigger puzzle that now makes sense.

This lens doesn't make the pain easier, but it makes it less confusing. You're not broken. You're not crazy. Your nervous system learned something, and it can learn something else. That's not just hope. That's the mechanism.

Change is possible, but it requires patience. The nervous system didn't get stuck overnight, and it won't unstick overnight either. Progress may be slow, nonlinear, and sometimes frustrating. There will be setbacks. There will be days when the old patterns feel insurmountable. But each slight shift in how you move, sleep, think, or regulate stress is a signal to your nervous system that safety is possible. And over time, those signals accumulate.

You don't need to believe in miracles. You need to understand that your system is plastic. That which was learned can be unlearned. Those small, consistent inputs, repeated over time, can reshape pathways that feel permanent. The road is long, but it's there. And now you have a map.

Looking Ahead

The following section will move from theory into practice. If maladaptive neuroplasticity explains why pain persists, then new inputs and new experiences can explain how it changes. Section Three will explore the tools: movement, sleep, nervous system regulation, pacing, and more. We'll look at how applying them through this lens can help the nervous system redraw its maps and relearn safety. This is where understanding becomes action.

Endnotes

[1] Nijs, J., Leysen, L., Vanlauwe, J., Logghe, T., Ickmans, K., Polli, A., Malfliet, A., Coppieters, I., & Huysmans, E. (2019). Treatment of central sensitization in patients with chronic pain: Time for change? *Expert Opinion on Pharmacotherapy*, 20(16), 1961–1970.

[2] Moseley, G. L., & Flor, H. (2012). Targeting cortical representations in the treatment of chronic pain: A review. *Neurorehabilitation and Neural Repair*, 26(6), 646–652.

[3] Finan, P. H., Goodin, B. R., & Smith, M. T. (2013). The association of sleep and pain: An update and a path forward. *The Journal of Pain*, 14(12), 1539–1552.

[4] Hannibal, K. E., & Bishop, M. D. (2014). Chronic stress, cortisol dysfunction, and pain: A psychoneuroendocrine rationale for stress management in pain rehabilitation. *Physical Therapy*, 94(12), 1816–1825.

[5] Bialosky, J. E., Bishop, M. D., Price, D. D., Robinson, M. E., & George, S. Z. (2009). The mechanisms of manual therapy in the treatment of musculoskeletal pain: A comprehensive model. *Manual Therapy*, 14(5), 531–538.

CHAPTER EIGHT

Movement As Medicine

Before we go further, I want to clear something up.

My background is in massage therapy and personal training. Not the relaxation spa kind of massage. I worked strictly in sports and pain management. On the training side, my focus was on strength and conditioning for athletes. I've done some work in aesthetics, but mostly my focus is on building performance. That's where I first learned about concepts like scaling and progressive overload, the principle that the body adapts best when challenges are introduced gradually.

I'm not saying you have to become an athlete. I'm not asking you to live that lifestyle or adopt their routines. What I've realized over years of working with people in pain is that the same principles apply, just with a completely different starting point and application. The difference is in how they look and where you start.

For an athlete, progression might mean adding weight to a barbell. For you, it might mean standing from a chair one extra time, or walking to the mailbox instead of the driveway. The principle is identical. The application is unique. And your goals are your own.

Because I understand both exercise science and maladaptive neuroplasticity, I've come to believe many traditional exercise modalities may have failed you in the past, not because movement itself was wrong, but because the approach didn't fit the state of your nervous system. Altering how we apply these principles is far more important than abandoning them altogether.

I've had multiple clients who went through physical therapy, worked hard, followed the protocol exactly as they were told, and ended up worse. One woman came to me after three rounds of PT for fibromyalgia. Each time, she was given a program with a higher frequency and intensity than her body could tolerate. It didn't matter that she was flaring after every session. The protocol was the protocol. The problem wasn't the exercises themselves. It was that they threw way too much stimulus at her nervous system all at once.

When she finally found a PT who understood nervous system sensitivity, everything changed. They reduced both frequency and intensity, and found the right amount of stimulus to work within her nervous system's thresholds without constantly lighting her up. And for the first time in years, she started making progress. Not because she'd suddenly "gotten stronger" in the traditional sense, but because her nervous system had learned that movement was safe.

This isn't just a physical therapy problem. I've had clients who went to personal trainers who pushed them through bootcamp-style sessions because "everyone else can handle it." I've had clients who went to massage therapists who worked too deeply, chasing some outdated idea that "deep tissue" means digging in as hard as possible, leaving them flared up for days. Then their doctors told them fibro patients can't handle deep work, which isn't true. What fibro patients can't handle is mindless deep work. When I worked with these same clients, focusing on tissue engagement rather than depth for its own sake, restoring balance and function rather than just mashing into tight spots, they actually improved.

I say this not to position myself as the one practitioner who "gets it," but to make a point: the issue isn't the modality. It's the approach. Physical therapy works when it's applied with nervous system sensitivity. Personal training works when it's scaled appropriately. Massage therapy works when it's intelligent, not aggressive. The problem is systemic. Too many practitioners are working from protocols designed for people whose nervous systems aren't already stuck in overdrive. And when those protocols fail, patients are told they're the problem. They're not. The approach is.

So what's the alternative? If traditional protocols don't fit, what does?

Why Movement Works

In Chapter 2, we discussed how movement updates cortical maps, interrupts pain loops, and teaches the nervous system that threat signals are false alarms. But knowing why movement helps doesn't make it less terrifying when you're the one in pain. This chapter is about the how.

How to move when movement itself feels like the enemy.

Movement is more than exercise. It's input. It sends signals to the brain about what the body can do, what it can't, and, most importantly, what's safe to try again. When pain signals have become noisy and confused, movement can act as a cleaner, healthier signal. Over time, these signals retrain the brain's maps and help overwrite maladaptive patterns.[1]

A comprehensive review of research found that physical activity and exercise can reduce pain severity and improve physical function in adults with chronic pain. However, the effects vary by condition and individual.[2] This is why movement is medicine.

This approach isn't new. Researchers have been proving it for years. Daniel Clauw has published extensively on fibromyalgia and central sensitization, highlighting the importance of careful, graded activity as a foundation for treatment.[3] Ginevra Liptan, in *The FibroManual*, emphasizes pacing and nervous-system-sensitive exercise, offering clear guidance on how patients can scale activity without provoking endless flares.[4] Andrea Furlan's work underscores the value of safe, graded activity and pacing strategies for chronic pain, teaching patients and providers alike how to apply these principles in daily life.[5]

Together, their work validates the same idea. You're not imagining your pain, and you're not broken. The nervous system learns through repetition. Give it consistent, safe input, and it retrains itself. This is the heart of movement as medicine.

The Fear You're Not Talking About

Most people with chronic pain don't avoid movement because they don't understand its benefits. They avoid it because they're terrified.

Terrified it will cause a flare. Terrified that pain during movement means they're causing damage. Fearful that their body is so broken that even gentle exercise will make things worse.

And that fear isn't irrational. You've probably experienced it before. You felt okay, decided to go for a walk or do some stretching, and then spent the next three days in bed, unable to move. Your nervous system learned from that experience. It learned that movement equals danger.

But here's what actually happened: you didn't damage anything. You triggered your nervous system's alarm, and it responded by amplifying pain signals to try to protect you.[6] The tissue was fine. The threat detection system was doing its job badly.

As we covered in Chapter 2, this is the difference between hurt and harm. The pain was real. The threat wasn't. But your nervous system doesn't know that yet. It's operating on old information, outdated maps, and a hair-trigger alarm system that fires at the slightest provocation.

The problem is that fear-based avoidance makes everything worse. When you stop moving, your muscles weaken, your joints stiffen, and your brain's body map becomes even more blurred.[7] The less you move, the more the brain interprets any attempt to move as a threat. The map loses definition. The system forgets what normal movement feels like.

It's a vicious cycle. And the only way out is through.

But "through" doesn't mean pushing through pain recklessly. It means teaching your nervous system, through repeated safe experiences, that the threat it's perceiving isn't real. It means starting so small that the alarm doesn't trip. And then building from there, gradually, consistently, until movement stops feeling like danger.

This is what decades of research on fear-avoidance have shown.[8] Fear of movement is often a bigger predictor of disability than the pain itself. The fear keeps you stuck. The avoidance reinforces the fear. And the cycle deepens until movement feels impossible.

Breaking that cycle starts with understanding that movement, done right, isn't the enemy. It's the way forward.

Pacing: The Inconvenient Solution

Most people with chronic pain fall into one of two patterns.

The first is the push-crash cycle. You feel okay, so you do everything you've been putting off. You clean the house, run errands, and maybe even exercise. Then you pay for it with days or weeks of increased pain. You crash hard, rest until you feel better, and repeat the cycle.

The second is fear-avoidance. You avoid movement entirely because you're terrified of making things worse. You rest constantly, hoping the pain will go away on its own. But it doesn't. And when you finally do try to move, even small efforts feel overwhelming because your system has deconditioned and become hypersensitive.

Both patterns reinforce the problem. The push-crash cycle teaches your nervous system that activity equals danger. Fear-avoidance leads to deconditioning, which makes everything harder and more painful when you do try to move.

The solution is pacing, finding a sustainable middle ground, and sticking to it even when you feel good.

Pacing means setting a baseline of activity that you can do consistently, even on bad days. It means slowly, ridiculously slowly, increasing that baseline. We're talking 5-10% increases over weeks, not days.[9] And it means resisting the urge to do more just because you feel better.

This is where most people struggle. When you have a good day, the temptation is to capitalize on it. To catch up on everything you've been unable to do. But doing too much on a good day often triggers a flare, which reinforces the nervous system's belief that activity is dangerous. You're back to square one.

Pacing asks you to do less than you think you can, even when you feel good. It feels like taking a step backward when all you want is to feel normal again. It's frustrating. It's slow. And it doesn't feel like progress in the moment.

But this is how you retrain your nervous system to trust movement. You show it, through repeated consistent experiences, that activity within your threshold doesn't lead to disaster. Over time, the threshold shifts. What was once hard becomes manageable. And you can build from there.

The truth about pacing is that it works. But it requires patience that most people don't feel like they have. You've been in pain for months or years. You want relief now. But the nervous system doesn't respond to desperation. It responds to consistency.

Graded Exposure: Teaching Your Brain It's Safe

Graded exposure is a technique borrowed from anxiety treatment, and it works just as well for pain.[10]

The idea is simple: start with movements or activities that cause minimal pain or fear, and gradually work up to more challenging ones. The key is that each step should feel manageable. Uncomfortable, maybe, but not overwhelming.

If walking is painful, start with standing for two minutes. If lifting your arm overhead hurts, start with lifting it halfway. If exercise feels impossible, start with gentle stretching or even just moving your joints through their range of motion while lying down.

The goal isn't to push through pain. The goal is to show your nervous system that movement doesn't equal harm. Over time, with consistent exposure to safe movement, the alarm system gradually quiets.

Let's say you haven't been able to reach overhead for 2 years due to shoulder pain. Every time you tried, the pain was so intense you'd stop immediately. Your doctor told you that you have a rotator cuff issue, but imaging showed nothing significant. The tissue wasn't the problem. The nervous system was.

So you start with your arm at your side, just lifting it forward a few inches. No pain. You hold that range for a week, practicing twice a day. Then you add a few more inches. Still manageable. Week by week, you increase the range, always staying within a tolerable threshold. After months, you can reach overhead again. Not because the rotator cuff healed, but because your brain learned that the movement was safe.

This is graded exposure. You're not forcing your way through pain. You're teaching your nervous system, one small step at a time, that the movements you've been avoiding are actually safe.

Research supports this approach across chronic pain conditions.[11] The brain updates its maps based on experience. Give it repeated safe experiences, and it rewrites the story. The movement that once felt dangerous becomes neutral, then easy, then automatic.

Why Small Movements Matter

A common misconception is that if movement hurts or flares symptoms, it should be avoided. The truth is more nuanced. Flares often mean the nervous system has been overloaded, not that the movement itself is dangerous. The solution is not avoidance, but scaling.

The goal is to find the version of a movement that challenges the system without overwhelming it, then repeat it consistently so the brain relearns safety.[12]

You might notice that squatting always leads to flare-ups. Your conclusion is never to do a squat. But the real issue wasn't that squatting was unsafe. It was that your nervous system was unprepared for that position. Just as an athlete who struggles at the bottom of a squat might work isometrically in that weak spot, you may need to practice scaled squats from a chair or barstool at a frequency and range your body can handle.

Over time, the nervous system adapts. The flare is not the enemy. It's feedback that the load was too much, just like an athlete who maxes out too often. The principle is the same, scaled down.

Pain neuroscience education combined with graded motor imagery has been shown to reduce pain and improve function in chronic pain conditions by retraining the brain to perceive movement as safe.[13]

Small movements work because they bypass the alarm system. Your brain doesn't perceive them as threats. And when you repeat them consistently, the brain starts to believe that this area of the body, this movement pattern, is safe. The cortical map clears. The pain pathway weakens. The system recalibrates.

This is why you can't skip steps. You can't go from avoiding squats to doing full-depth squats and expect your nervous system to be okay with it. That's like jumping into the deep end when you're still learning to swim. You'll panic. The alarm will fire. And you'll reinforce the very pattern you're trying to break.

Start small. Stay small until it's easy. Then build.

Scaling and Progressive Overload

In athletic training, progressive overload means gradually increasing volume or intensity to build strength. The same principle applies here, but with a different starting point.[14]

Here's the thing: many therapists are trained with the idea that there's a standard baseline, a so-called bottom end, from which people in therapy should begin. Those baselines were written for the average person without a nervous system already shaped by maladaptive neuroplasticity. For people living with fibro or other chronic pain conditions, that standard baseline often doesn't apply.

This doesn't mean you are weak or less than. It means you are beginning from a different place than what practitioners were taught to expect. Respecting that difference is essential.

For some, the right entry point might be one set of two or three chair squats once a week. For others, isometric holds in the position they fear most. As these become easier, progress comes either from more repetitions or more frequent practice, like spreading out free-throw practice across the week instead of doing all 300 shots in one day.

Consistency and repetition matter more than intensity. That's a tough sell for anyone who grew up believing "no pain, no gain." But if your system is already on high alert, intensity doesn't build. It breaks. The goal is to teach the nervous system that movement is safe, not to prove how much you can endure.

Let me give you some context from the training side. When I program for athletes, I would never have them work at 90-100% of their max every workout. That's not how you build strength. It's how you break someone. Most training volume sits in the 70-80% range, challenging but not overtaxing. Even when programs push toward and even above 90%, those sets account for only a tiny percentage of the overall volume. The vast majority of the work happens in a range that's manageable, repeatable, and sustainable.

If I had an athlete train at 95% of their max every set, every rep, I would break them. Quickly. Their nervous system couldn't recover. Their joints would give out. Their performance would tank.

It's no different here. Pushing every workout to the limit, hoping that someone with fibro will "catch up," isn't training. It's destruction. Taxing their nervous system by pushing every session to the extreme is the same as having an athlete max out daily. It doesn't build resilience. It reinforces the threat response.

This is why most movement interventions fall short. They apply protocols designed for people whose nervous systems can handle higher intensity volume. But if your baseline is already sensitized, that approach doesn't work. It backfires. The 5-10% increases over the course of weeks might seem painfully slow, but it's the same principle I'd use with any athlete. You build capacity gradually, respecting the system's current threshold, so the adaptations stick.

Consider a fibro patient starting with two-chair squats twice a week. After a month, it's three squats twice a week. After two months, it's three squats three times a week. After three months, it's five squats three times a week. The progression is glacial. But by month six, they're doing ten squats without flaring. A year in, they're doing bodyweight squats from a standing position.

That's not because they got stronger in the traditional sense. It's because their nervous system learned, through hundreds of repetitions at tolerable doses, that squatting is safe.

This is the power of scaling. You meet the nervous system where it is, not where you wish it were. And you build from there, patiently, consistently, trusting that small inputs add up over time.

What Flares Actually Mean

Let's talk about flares because they're going to happen. And when they do, you need to know how to interpret them.

A flare doesn't mean you failed. It doesn't mean you damaged your body. And it doesn't erase all the progress you've made.

A flare is feedback. It shows you where your nervous system's edge is today. And edges can shift over time.

You may have pushed a little too hard. Maybe you didn't sleep well the night before, and your system was already sensitized. Maybe you were stressed about something unrelated, which primed your nervous system to overreact. Flares are multifactorial. They're rarely about one thing.

The key is to interpret the flare as data, not disaster. What was different? What can you adjust next time? How long did the flare last compared to previous ones? Even if it feels the same, the recovery time can tell you whether your system is becoming more resilient.

Track it. Write it down. Look for patterns. Over time, you'll see that flares become shorter, less intense, or easier to manage. That's progress, even if it doesn't feel like it in the moment.

But let's be honest about something else. Some days, the feedback says, *Not today. Not this week.* And that's okay. Rest isn't the same as giving up. Your nervous system is doing something during that rest. It's processing, recalibrating, trying to make sense of the inputs you've given it. Trust that. You're not starting over every time you pause. You're allowing the system to catch up.

If you don't have access to a practitioner who gets this, you can still apply these principles on your own. Start small, track what flares you and what doesn't, and let the data guide you. You don't need permission to begin. You just need curiosity and patience.

Finding Your Personal Baseline

One of the most empowering steps you can take is identifying your own baseline. This means noticing what you can do without provoking a flare, even if it seems very small. For some, it may be standing from a chair once. For others, it might be a short walk to the end of the driveway. The point is not to measure yourself against anyone else, but to discover where your nervous system says, *this is tolerable right now*.

That baseline is your starting place, not a judgment of strength or weakness.

Your baseline is also dynamic. As you repeat safe inputs consistently, your system adapts and your baseline shifts. What was once difficult gradually becomes easy, and you can build from there. Scaling can then take many forms: adding repetition, practicing more frequently, slowing down a movement for more control, or adding variety. Because you understand where your baseline is, you are in control of how to scale.

Take a minute. What's one thing you can do right now, today, that doesn't light you up? That's your starting line.

It could be standing for thirty seconds. Maybe it's walking around the block. Perhaps it's lifting a can of soup overhead. Whatever it is, that's your baseline. Own it. Practice it. And when it becomes easy, add one small increment.

This is how you build trust with your body. Not through one big breakthrough, but through hundreds of small, successful experiences that teach your nervous system that movement is safe.

Putting It Together

Movement is medicine when it's scaled, repeated, and seen as input to the nervous system. It's not about pushing through pain or proving toughness. It's about finding the entry point that doesn't flare you up, repeating it often enough to retrain your brain, and progressing gradually so your system learns a new story about safety.

Over time, those small, manageable movements add up to strength, confidence, and freedom.

Again, think of it like tuning a radio. Right now, your nervous system is picking up static, noisy, confusing signals that make it hard to tell what's real and what's just interference. Small, consistent movement practice gradually clears the channel. You're not forcing the signal through. You're teaching the system to recognize it again.

What's one movement you've been avoiding because of fear of pain? How might you practice a smaller version of it safely and consistently, without overwhelming your system?

In the following chapters, we'll look at other inputs that reinforce this same principle: sleep, recovery, regulation, and trust. Movement retrains the map. But if you're not sleeping, if your nervous system is still stuck in fight-or-flight, that retraining can't stick. These pieces work together, and understanding how they connect is what makes the difference between spinning your wheels and actually moving forward.

But movement is where it starts. It's the first signal you send your brain that says, *"Maybe this body isn't broken after all."*

Endnotes

[1] Moseley, G. L., & Butler, D. S. (2015). Fifteen years of explaining pain: The past, present, and future. *Journal of Pain*, 16(9), 807–813.

[2] Geneen, L. J., Moore, R. A., Clarke, C., Martin, D., Colvin, L. A., & Smith, B. H. (2017). Physical activity and exercise for chronic pain in adults: An overview of Cochrane Reviews. *Cochrane Database of Systematic Reviews*, 4, CD011279.

[3] Clauw, D. J. (2014). Fibromyalgia: A clinical review. *JAMA*, 311(15), 1547–1555.

[4] Liptan, G. (2016). *The FibroManual: A Complete Fibromyalgia Treatment Guide for You and Your Doctor.* Ballantine Books.

[5] Furlan, A. D., Yazdi, F., Tsertsvadze, A., Gross, A., Van Tulder, M., Santaguida, L., Gagnier, J., Ammendolia, C.,

Dryden, T., & Doucette, S. (2010). A systematic review and meta-analysis of efficacy, cost-effectiveness, and safety of selected complementary and alternative medicine for neck and low-back pain. *Evidence-Based Complementary and Alternative Medicine*, 7(1), 95–113.

[6] Woolf, C. J. (2011). Central sensitization: Implications for the diagnosis and treatment of pain. *Pain*, 152(3 Suppl), S2-S15.

[7] Moseley, G. L., & Flor, H. (2012). Targeting cortical representations in the treatment of chronic pain: A review. *Neurorehabilitation and Neural Repair*, 26(6), 646-652.

[8] Vlaeyen, J. W., & Linton, S. J. (2012). Fear-avoidance model of chronic musculoskeletal pain: 12 years on. *Pain*, 153(6), 1144–1147.

[9] Antcliff, D., Keeley, P., Campbell, M., Oldham, J., & Woby, S. (2013). Activity pacing: Moving beyond the controversy to principles and practice. *Clinical Rehabilitation*, 27(12), 1099-1107.

[10] Vlaeyen, J. W., de Jong, J., Geilen, M., Heuts, P. H., & van Breukelen, G. (2001). Graded exposure in vivo in the treatment of pain-related fear: A replicated single-case experimental design in four patients with chronic low

back pain. *Behaviour Research and Therapy*, 39(2), 151-166.

[11] Vlaeyen, J. W. S., & Linton, S. J. (2012). Fear-avoidance model of chronic musculoskeletal pain: 12 years on. *Pain*, 153(6), 1144–1147.

[12] Nijs, J., Paul van Wilgen, C., Van Oosterwijck, J., van Ittersum, M., & Meeus, M. (2011). How to explain central sensitization to patients with 'unexplained' chronic musculoskeletal pain: Practice guidelines. *Manual Therapy*, 16(5), 413-418.

[13] Moseley, G. L. (2006). Graded motor imagery for pathologic pain: A randomized controlled trial. *Neurology*, 67(12), 2129-2134.

[14] Booth, J., Moseley, G. L., Schiltenwolf, M., Cashin, A., Davies, M., & Hübscher, M. (2017). Exercise for chronic musculoskeletal pain: A biopsychosocial approach. *Musculoskeletal Care*, 15(4), 413–421.

CHAPTER NINE

Sleep, Safety, and Foundations of Rest

Sleep and recovery are not luxuries. They are the foundations of healing. For people living with chronic pain, this is often the most frustrating advice they've ever heard. "Just get more sleep" or "sleep better" is the kind of empty guidance many have been given for years, without any explanation of *how* to do so. This chapter will cut through the noise. It will explain why sleep matters and how the nervous system can get stuck in overdrive. And it will discuss what practical tools can help bring it back toward recovery.

In Chapter 8, we covered movement as medicine, how to retrain your nervous system through graduated, safe inputs. But here's the reality. If you're not sleeping, those movement gains won't stick. Without it, you're trying to build on quicksand.

Why Sleep Matters for Pain

Sleep is when the nervous system recalibrates. During deep stages of rest, the brain processes signals and consolidates learning. This is where it also restores balance. Without it, the pain system becomes more sensitive. Research shows that poor or fragmented sleep lowers pain thresholds, increases inflammation, and increases the likelihood of flare-ups.[1] In simple terms: a tired nervous system is an irritable nervous system.

You can think of sleep as the body's nightly reset button. When the reset doesn't happen, the system boots up glitchy. Alarms misfire, and signals get confused. Everything feels harder the next day. For people with chronic pain, this vicious cycle becomes familiar. Pain disrupts sleep, and poor sleep amplifies pain.

For example, someone might find themselves tossing and turning for hours, jaw clenched, replaying stressful thoughts from the day. Their partner sleeps soundly beside them, but they're stuck in a loop. Instead of resting, they're rehashing conversations, worrying about tomorrow's tasks, and feeling their pain intensify with each passing hour. But by introducing a short journaling routine before bed, just five minutes of dumping thoughts onto paper, they create an outlet. The thoughts are still there, but they're no longer *inside*. Within two weeks, they're falling asleep in 20 minutes instead of 2 hours. The pain the next day is lighter. Not gone, but manageable. This demonstrates how small changes can alter how the brain prepares for rest.

Sleep Architecture: What Actually Happens When You Rest

To understand why sleep is so critical for pain, you need to understand what sleep actually does. Sleep isn't just one state; it's a carefully orchestrated cycle of stages, each with specific functions. When chronic pain disrupts this cycle, the body loses access to the very processes that could help it heal.

Stage 1 (N1): Light Sleep

This is the transition stage, the boundary between waking and sleeping. Your muscles relax, and your heart rate slows slightly. Your brain begins to disengage from external stimuli. You're easy to wake during this stage. This is as deep as sleep gets often for people with chronic pain whose nervous systems never fully let go.

Stage 2 (N2): Deeper Light Sleep

Brain activity slows further. Body temperature drops. This stage makes up about half of total sleep time in healthy sleepers. It's restorative, but not profoundly so. Think of it as maintenance mode, not complete repair.

Stage 3 (N3): Deep Sleep (Slow-Wave Sleep)

This is where the real work happens. During deep sleep, the brain releases growth hormone, which supports tissue repair and immune function.[2] Blood flow to muscles increases. The glymphatic system, the brain's waste-clearance system, becomes more active, flushing out metabolic byproducts that accumulated during the day.[3] Pain thresholds reset. Inhibitory pathways strengthen.

Without adequate deep sleep, the body can't complete these processes. The pain system stays sensitized. The immune system stays on alert. The brain's maps don't update properly.

REM Sleep: Rapid Eye Movement

For someone retraining their nervous system through movement or graded exposure, REM sleep is when those new patterns get encoded. This is when the brain processes emotions. It's where memories are consolidated, and learning is integrated. It's also when the brain sorts through emotional experiences, which is why REM deprivation often leads to increased anxiety and emotional reactivity.[4]

In chronic pain, sympathetic dominance keeps you cycling through Stages 1 and 2, never dropping into the deep, restorative stages. You might be in bed for eight hours, but your body only gets two hours of actual recovery. That's why you wake up exhausted, feeling like you were hit by a truck overnight. The system never got to reset.

The Pain-Sleep-Pain Cycle

Here's how the cycle works, and why it's so hard to break:

Pain disrupts sleep. When you're in pain, your body stays in sympathetic dominance. Muscles stay tense. The brain stays alert, scanning for threats. You don't drop into deep sleep because the nervous system interprets pain as a threat, which means staying vigilant.

Poor sleep amplifies pain. When you don't get enough deep sleep, your pain threshold drops. Studies show that even one night of poor sleep can increase pain sensitivity the next day by as much as 25%.[5] Your nervous system becomes more reactive. Signals that would have been tolerable yesterday feel sharper today.

Increased pain further disrupts sleep. Now you're dealing with heightened pain during the day, which makes it even harder to relax at night. The cycle tightens.

Nocturnal pain spikes compound the problem. Many people with chronic pain notice that pain feels worse at night, particularly around 3-4 AM. This isn't random. Cortisol, the hormone that helps modulate pain, naturally dips during the early morning hours. Without that buffer, pain signals come through louder.[6] You wake up, and the sleep cycle breaks. Even if you fall back asleep, you've missed the deep sleep window.

Medication timing matters. If you're taking pain medication, the timing can either support or sabotage sleep. Medications that wear off in the middle of the night can trigger waking. Medications that cause drowsiness but don't actually improve sleep quality leave you groggy, not rested. And some pain medications disrupt REM sleep, preventing the emotional and cognitive processing that happens during that stage.

This cycle doesn't break on its own. It requires deliberate intervention. And that intervention starts with understanding the nervous system's two operating modes.

Sympathetic vs. Parasympathetic: The Balance of Rest

As we discussed in Chapters 2 and 3, the nervous system has two modes: sympathetic (fight-or-flight) and parasympathetic (rest-and-repair). In chronic pain, sympathetic dominance becomes the default. Here's how that shows up in sleep:

Sympathetic dominance keeps the system on high alert. Heart rate stays elevated. Muscles stay tense. Digestion slows. The brain scans for danger. It's like a smoke detector going off all night. The alarms are blaring, but there is no real fire.

Parasympathetic dominance allows the body to downshift. Resources are directed toward healing. Heart rate slows. Breathing deepens. The repair crew finally comes in once the alarms are quiet.

Many people with chronic pain live in sympathetic dominance around the clock. Their nervous system interprets almost everything as a threat, even when no immediate danger exists.[7] It's like running a generator nonstop with no off switch. The motor screams, fuel burns, heat builds, and nothing ever gets to rest.

The goal isn't to eliminate the sympathetic response. It's to restore balance. To teach the system that it's safe to shift into parasympathetic mode at night, even if pain is still present.

Safety as a Foundation for Rest

Sleep and recovery aren't just about closing your eyes. They depend on cues of safety. The limbic system, which we explored in Chapter 3, has to be convinced that it's okay to relax.[8] Predictable routines, calming rituals, and signals of safety reduce background noise and let the system settle.

Safety can be both physical and emotional:

Physical safety might mean a dark, quiet environment, with comfortable bedding, and a consistent temperature. Each of these cues tells the body that nothing is threatening it physically, allowing the repair processes to activate.

Emotional safety comes from winding down rituals and predictable routines. These provide cues that tell the nervous system "you're safe now." For some, this may include reading a comforting book. For others, it may be prayer, meditation, or listening to familiar music. The key is repetition. When these safety inputs are repeated, the nervous system begins to shift its default from constant vigilance to a state in which repair is possible.

Consider someone who feels uneasy in complete darkness. Every creak of the house, every shift of shadow becomes a potential threat. Their heart rate remains elevated, and their muscles remain tight. Sleep remains elusive. They start by leaving a dim lamp on and playing soft background noise, such as rain sounds or white noise. Anything consistent. It feels like a small defeat at first, like they're "giving in" to fear. But within a week, their body begins to trust the environment. The sounds become predictable. The soft light becomes a signal: *this is safe*. Over time, as trust builds, they might gradually transition to darker conditions. But the lesson isn't about forcing themselves into darkness. It's about recognizing that emotional safety can be just as important as physical comfort.

Tools for Better Sleep & Recovery

Here are practical ways to reinforce parasympathetic dominance and improve rest:

1. Environment

A cool, dark, and quiet room signals physical safety.[9] Blackout curtains or an eye mask block intrusive light, while white noise can cover inconsistent sounds. Supportive bedding and proper airflow can also make a difference. Temperature matters more than most people realize. The body's core temperature naturally drops during sleep as part of the parasympathetic shift. Cooler skin signals to the brain that it's time to rest. A room that's too warm disrupts this process, keeping the nervous system slightly activated. Research suggests aiming for a range of 60-67°F (15-19°C). If that feels too cold initially, start warmer and gradually adjust. In all fairness, though, most sleep research is done in controlled lab environments. Not in hot, humid climates with real electric bills. Cooler temperatures support deeper sleep, but that doesn't mean you need to set your thermostat to 60°F. Simply lowering the temperature a few degrees from your daytime setting, or creating a cooler sleep environment with fans, breathable bedding, or light airflow, can achieve the same effect without wrecking your utility bill.

Consider someone who's been struggling with sleep for years. They've tried everything: meditation, supplements, and new mattresses. Nothing helped. Then they lower their bedroom temperature from 72°F to 69°F and start using a fan for white noise. Within two weeks, they're sleeping five hours straight instead of waking every hour. The change isn't dramatic or complicated. It's just giving the nervous system the environmental cues it needs to believe rest is safe.

Reflection prompt: What's one small change you could make to your sleep environment this week? A cooler room, a darker space, or calmer sound? Pick one and try it for three nights.

2. Pre-Sleep Rituals

Gentle breathing exercises, such as slow inhales for 4 seconds and exhales for 6 seconds, can shift the body into parasympathetic mode.[10] The extended exhale is key. It activates the vagus nerve and signals safety to the brain.

Progressive relaxation, scanning through each muscle group and consciously releasing tension, teaches the brain that it's okay to let go. Start at the top of the head. Notice any tension in the forehead, the jaw, or the neck. Don't force anything to relax; just observe it, then move down. Shoulders, arms, chest, abdomen. Keep going until you reach your toes. The practice isn't about achieving perfect relaxation. It's about building awareness of what tension feels like, and giving your body permission to release it.

Journaling briefly before bed offloads anxious thoughts, making space for calm. This doesn't need to be formal or profound. It's just a brain dump. Three things that happened today. One thing you're worried about. One thing that went okay. Getting it out of your head and onto paper creates separation.

Other variations include stretching, warm showers, or guided audio recordings. Avoiding heavy meals, caffeine, and screens reduces stimulation. These practices create a consistent pre-sleep script, teaching the nervous system that it's safe to power down.

Reflection prompt: Which ritual could you add tonight that would signal safety to your system?

3. The Role of Touch and Bodywork

For some people, gentle bodywork before bed can be a powerful pre-sleep signal. A brief self-massage on the hands, feet, neck, or wherever tension holds can help the nervous system downshift. The pressure doesn't need to be deep; even light, intentional touch can signal safety.

If you have access to a skilled manual therapist who understands chronic pain or hypermobility, a calming session can be part of your routine. Many clients over the years have reported better sleep the first few nights after a session. The goal isn't aggressive "deep tissue" work for its own sake. It's about engagement, response, and helping the body recognize that it's okay to let go.

We'll explore manual therapy in much greater depth in the next chapter, including how it works as a nervous system recalibration tool, what to look for in a therapist, and self-release techniques you can use daily.

4. Building Calm Throughout the Day

Sleep doesn't begin when your head hits the pillow. It starts with how you manage your nervous system throughout the day. If you run at full throttle from morning to night, expecting the system to shut down entirely at bedtime is unrealistic. But if you build in small moments of downshift, such as a two-minute breathing break at lunch, a short walk after sitting for an hour, or a pause to stretch before starting the next task, you're teaching the system that it doesn't have to be in overdrive all the time. Those small deposits make withdrawal at night easier.

We'll explore daily regulation practices in greater depth in the next chapter. For now, know that the calmer your nervous system is during the day, the easier it is to rest at night.

Reflection prompt: How might you add one downshift into your day tomorrow?

5. Consistency Over Perfection

The immediate goal isn't eight flawless hours, but steady signals of safety. Minor improvements in sleep quality or duration accumulate over time, gradually reducing pain sensitivity. Consistency helps retrain the nervous system, just as repetition builds muscle. Keeping the same sleep and wake times each day reinforces circadian rhythm stability and reduces the restlessness that shows up when the system doesn't know what to expect.[11] Morning light exposure and routine cues further strengthen this rhythm.

Some nights will be better than others. That's expected. The win isn't "perfect sleep every night." It's "more nights trending toward better sleep than a month ago." Track the pattern, not the individual night.

Consider someone who's been sleeping poorly for over a decade. They start with one change, perhaps going to bed at 10 PM every night, even on weekends. For the first month, nothing seems different. They're still awake until midnight most nights. But they keep the routine. By month two, they notice they're getting drowsy around 10:30 PM. By month three, they're asleep by 11 PM most nights. By month six, they're sleeping six hours straight and waking up less exhausted. It isn't fast. It isn't dramatic. But it works because of consistency.

Reflection prompt

Which part of your schedule could you make more consistent?

Supplements That May Support Sleep

Lifestyle changes are always the foundation, but some supplements can provide gentle support. These are not cures, and they work best alongside consistent routines, environmental changes, and emotional safety cues. Always consult a healthcare provider before taking them, especially if you're taking other medications or have underlying health conditions.

Magnesium: Plays a role in muscle relaxation and calming the nervous system. Many people with chronic pain or EDS find that magnesium can reduce nighttime tension and support deeper sleep.[12] Magnesium glycinate is often better tolerated than other forms and may have the added benefit of the glycine component. Typical dosing ranges from 200-400mg before bed, but start low and adjust based on response and tolerance.

Glycine: An amino acid that may improve sleep onset and quality. It supports nervous system regulation and is sometimes used for connective tissue health as well.[13] Studies suggest 3 grams before bed can improve subjective sleep quality and reduce daytime fatigue. It's generally well-tolerated and can be taken alone or as part of magnesium glycinate.

Melatonin: Helps regulate circadian rhythms, especially for those with disrupted schedules or delayed sleep cycles.[14] However, recent research has raised concerns about potential downsides to melatonin use. These include hormonal effects, dependency, rebound insomnia, and inconsistent dosing in over-the-counter supplements. If you're considering melatonin, do thorough research and consult with a healthcare provider before starting. If you do use it, start with a low dose (0.5-1mg) about an hour before bed, rather than the higher doses often sold commercially. More isn't better with melatonin. It's about timing and consistency.

These tools should be seen as supportive, not primary interventions. They can't fix a chaotic sleep environment, an overactive nervous system running on caffeine at 8 PM, or a lack of safety cues. But when combined with the foundational practices above, they can make the shift toward parasympathetic dominance easier.

When Nothing Seems to Work

Let's address the elephant in the room. You've tried everything. You've adjusted your environment, established routines, taken supplements, and practiced breathing exercises. And you're still not sleeping. Or you're sleeping, but you're waking up just as exhausted.

This can be incredibly frustrating. And it's not uncommon.

If you've been consistent with sleep hygiene for three months and you're still struggling, it's worth considering a few possibilities:

Underlying sleep disorders. Conditions like sleep apnea, restless leg syndrome, or periodic limb movement disorder can sabotage sleep quality even when you're doing everything right. A sleep study can identify these issues. Sleep apnea, in particular, is often undiagnosed in people with chronic pain and can significantly worsen pain sensitivity.[15]

Cognitive-behavioral therapy for insomnia (CBT-I). This is an evidence-based treatment that addresses the thought patterns and behaviors that perpetuate insomnia. It's not just "think positive." It's a structured, targeted intervention that helps retrain the brain's relationship with sleep. Research shows CBT-I is often more effective than medication for long-term sleep improvement.[16]

Sleep restriction paradox. This sounds counterintuitive. But sometimes spending less time in bed actually improves sleep. If you're in bed for 10 hours but only sleep 4, your brain starts to associate the bed with wakefulness. Sleep restriction therapy involves limiting time in bed to match the actual amount of sleep. Then it gradually increases as sleep efficiency improves. This should be done under the guidance of a sleep specialist.

Medication may be necessary for the short term. This isn't failure. If your nervous system is so dysregulated that you can't access sleep at all, short-term medication can provide a window for other interventions to take hold. The goal isn't long-term dependency. It's stabilization.

The point is this: if you've tried everything in this chapter and you're still not sleeping, you're not broken. You may need more specialized help. And that's okay.

Consider someone who's tried everything in this chapter for two years. They tried every supplement, every routine, every environmental change. Nothing works. They finally see a sleep specialist who discovers moderate sleep apnea. Once they start using a CPAP machine, their sleep improves within weeks. Their pain levels drop within a month. The problem wasn't that they weren't trying hard enough. The problem was an underlying condition that needed to be addressed.

Don't suffer in silence. If sleep remains elusive despite your best efforts, seek specialized evaluation.

Putting It Together: The Sleep Foundation

Sleep isn't a switch you flip. It's a process you build with every cue of safety. Every pre-sleep ritual, and every consistent bedtime, is a signal to your nervous system: *It's okay to rest. You're safe here.*

Some of these changes will feel small. Adjusting the temperature. Dimming the lights an hour earlier. Writing three sentences in a journal. They might not seem like enough, especially when you're dealing with years of poor sleep and chronic pain. But small, consistent inputs reshape the nervous system over time. That's not hopeful thinking, that's neuroplasticity.

Take someone who's been struggling with sleep for five years. They might start with just one change, such as going to bed at the same time every night, even on weekends. It feels pointless at first. They're still awake for hours, staring at the ceiling. But after two weeks, they notice they're getting drowsy around that time. Even if they don't fall asleep immediately, they add a second change. Journaling for five minutes before bed. A week later, they're asleep within forty minutes instead of two hours. The pain the next day is still there, but it's not as sharp. Three months in, they're sleeping six hours most nights instead of three. That's not a cure. That's recalibration in action.

The nervous system learns through repetition. If you repeat inconsistent schedules and high stimulation before bed, it learns to expect chaos. Especially with no wind-down rituals. But. If you repeat consistent routines and calming inputs, it learns to expect safety. The key is giving it predictable cues. And when it expects safety, it can finally rest.

That's what this chapter is about. Not perfection. Not a cure. But recalibration, one small input at a time.

In the next chapter, we'll build on this foundation by exploring daily nervous system recalibration, which are the active skills and practices that teach your system how to regulate throughout the day, making nighttime rest not just possible, but easier.

Endnotes

[1] Finan, P. H., Goodin, B. R., & Smith, M. T. (2013). The association of sleep and pain: An update and a path forward. *Journal of Pain*, 14(12), 1539–1552.

[2] Van Cauter, E., & Plat, L. (1996). Physiology of growth hormone secretion during sleep. *Journal of Pediatrics*, 128(5 Pt 2), S32–S37.

[3] Iliff, J. J., et al. (2012). A paravascular pathway facilitates CSF flow through the brain parenchyma and the clearance of interstitial solutes, including amyloid β. *Science Translational Medicine*, 4(147), 147ra111.

[4] Walker, M. P. (2009). The role of sleep in cognition and emotion. *Annals of the New York Academy of Sciences*, 1156(1), 168–197.

[5] Roehrs, T., Hyde, M., Blaisdell, B., Greenwald, M., & Roth, T. (2006). Sleep loss and REM sleep loss are hyperalgesic. *Sleep*, 29(2), 145–151.

[6] Born, J., Hansen, K., Marshall, L., Mölle, M., & Fehm, H. L. (1999). Timing the end of nocturnal sleep. *Nature*, 397(6714), 29–30.

[7] Borsook, D., Maleki, N., Becerra, L., & McEwen, B. (2012). Understanding migraine through the lens of maladaptive stress responses: A model disease of allostatic load. *Neuron*, 73(2), 219–234.

[8] Porges, S. W. (2011). *The Polyvagal Theory: Neurophysiological Foundations of Emotions, Attachment, Communication, and Self-regulation*. W. W. Norton & Company.

[9] Okamoto-Mizuno, K., & Mizuno, K. (2012). Effects of thermal environment on sleep and circadian rhythm. *Journal of Physiological Anthropology*, 31(1), 14.

[10] Jerath, R., Edry, J. W., Barnes, V. A., & Jerath, V. (2006). Physiology of long pranayamic breathing: Neural respiratory elements may provide a mechanism that explains how slow deep breathing shifts the

autonomic nervous system. *Medical Hypotheses*, 67(3), 566–571.

[11] Skeldon, A. C., Phillips, A. J., & Dijk, D. J. (2017). The effects of self-selected light-dark cycles and social constraints on human sleep and circadian timing: A modeling approach. *Scientific Reports*, 7, 45158.

[12] Abbasi, B., Kimiagar, M., Sadeghniiat, K., Shirazi, M. M., Hedayati, M., & Rashidkhani, B. (2012). The effect of magnesium supplementation on primary insomnia in elderly: A double-blind placebo-controlled clinical trial. *Journal of Research in Medical Sciences*, 17(12), 1161–1169.

[13] Bannai, M., & Kawai, N. (2012). New therapeutic strategy for amino acid medicine: Glycine improves the quality of sleep. *Journal of Pharmacological Sciences*, 118(2), 145–148.

[14] Sack, R. L., Auckley, D., Auger, R. R., Carskadon, M. A., Wright, K. P., Vitiello, M. V., Zhdanova, I. V., & The Standards of Practice Committee of the American Academy of Sleep Medicine. (2007). Circadian rhythm sleep disorders: Part II, advanced sleep phase disorder and delayed sleep phase disorder. *Sleep*, 30(11), 1484–1501.

[15] Smith, M. T., & Haythornthwaite, J. A. (2004). How do sleep disturbance and chronic pain inter-relate? Insights from the longitudinal and cognitive-behavioral clinical trials literature. *Sleep Medicine Reviews*, 8(2), 119–132.

[16] Trauer, J. M., Qian, M. Y., Doyle, J. S., Rajaratnam, S. M., & Cunnington, D. (2015). Cognitive behavioral therapy for chronic insomnia: A systematic review and meta-analysis. *Annals of Internal Medicine*, 163(3), 191–204.

CHAPTER TEN

Recovery Tools

BEYOND SLEEP

You've got the bricks. Everything we've covered so far, the science of pain, how your brain builds maps, and why sleep matters. Those are the foundational pieces. But bricks alone don't make a wall. You need mortar. Something to hold them together and create a structure that can actually stand.

This chapter is the mortar.

These are the practices that take everything you've learned and turn it into something functional. Something you can actually live with. Because understanding why you're in pain doesn't make the pain stop. But understanding *plus* consistent action? That's where recovery lives.

If you've started working on your sleep, really working on it, you've already done the most challenging part. You've given your nervous system the one thing it can't function without. But here's the reality no one tells you: sleep is necessary, but not sufficient. Your nervous system doesn't live in a vacuum. It responds to everything. Stress, movement, food, connection, touch.

And if those other inputs are still screaming "danger," sleep alone won't be enough to turn the volume down.

Your nervous system speaks multiple languages. It listens to your breath, your movement patterns, the food you eat, the people around you, and the hands that touch you. Each of these is a channel through which you can send the same essential message: *You're safe. You can stand down.*

Some of these channels will feel more accessible than others. Some will feel impossible, especially if you're deep in a flare. That's okay. The goal isn't perfection. It's consistency in whatever small doses you can manage.

Let's talk about how to use each channel.

The Language of Breath: Direct Communication

Your breath is the most direct line of communication you have with your autonomic nervous system. No other signal travels faster or more reliably.

As we discussed in Chapter 9, your nervous system operates in two modes: sympathetic (fight-or-flight) and parasympathetic (rest-and-digest). When you're stressed, your breathing becomes shallow and fast, primarily through the chest, which is driven by the sympathetic nervous system. When you're calm, your breathing shifts to your diaphragm, slow and deep, driven by the parasympathetic system.[1]

The beautiful part? This communication goes both ways. You can't always control your thoughts or your pain levels, but you can control your breath. And when you slow your breath down deliberately, you send a clear message to your nervous system: "We're safe. We can relax."[2]

Here's the uncomfortable truth most people don't want to hear. Stress doesn't just make pain worse. In many cases, chronic stress is what keeps the pain loop running.

When you're stressed, your body releases cortisol and adrenaline.[3] Your heart rate increases. Your muscles tense. Your brain shifts into high-alert mode, scanning for threats. And in that state, even normal sensations can feel dangerous.

Now imagine that stress response never shuts off. Maybe it started with a major trauma, physical or emotional. It may have built up slowly over years of pushing through while ignoring your body's signals, and trying to keep up with demands that never let up.

Either way, your nervous system learned to stay on guard.

And here's the kicker. Once your nervous system gets stuck in that loop, it doesn't matter if the original stressor is gone. The system itself becomes the stressor. The pain becomes the threat. And the cycle reinforces itself.

Breaking that cycle requires more than just "calming down" or "thinking positive." It requires deliberate practices that teach your nervous system it's safe to stand down.

Breathing as Reset

One technique many people find helpful is 4-7-8 breathing. Breathe in through your nose for 4 counts. Hold for 7 counts. Exhale slowly through your mouth for 8 counts.

Repeat that four times, and you'll likely notice a shift. Not dramatic, but real. Your heart rate slows. The tension in your shoulders eases slightly, and the static quiets.

Do this once a day, and it's a nice stress-relief tool. Do it multiple times throughout the day, especially when you notice tension building, and it starts to retrain your nervous system's baseline.

The point isn't to achieve some zen state. The point is to interrupt the loop. To give your nervous system one clear, undeniable signal that right now, in this moment, you're not actually under threat.

Systematic reviews have found that slow, controlled breathing activates the parasympathetic nervous system, reduces stress hormones, and can improve pain tolerance.[4]

Grounding When You're Spinning

Grounding is about bringing your awareness back to the present moment, away from the spiral of fear and catastrophizing that chronic pain loves to feed.

One simple practice you can implement is the 5-4-3-2-1 technique.[5] Name 5 things you can see. Name 4 things you can touch. Name 3 things you can hear. Name 2 things you can smell. Name 1 thing you can taste.

It sounds almost childish, but it works because it redirects your brain away from the threat circuits and into sensory processing. It reminds your nervous system that right now, in this moment, you're not in danger.

You can also use physical grounding. Press your feet into the floor. Feel the weight of your body in the chair. Run your hands under cold water. These simple sensory experiences interrupt the feedback loop.

Combining Breath and Movement

One practice that combines breath, movement, and grounding is qi gong. It's a Chinese movement practice that looks like slow-motion tai chi. It's made up of gentle, flowing movements coordinated with deep breathing. The beauty of qi gong is that it's explicitly designed to calm the nervous system, combining controlled breathing, focused attention, and gentle movement all at once.

YouTube has hundreds of free videos. Search "qi gong for beginners" or "qi gong for pain relief" and start with whatever feels manageable. But be careful. While it looks gentle and soft, it can actually be much more strenuous than it appears. I have had people report to me that they practiced for an entire hour the first time, leaving them wrecked afterward. Start for 5 or 10 minutes initially to test your tolerance here. But I highly suggest it, as this practice naturally bridges the breathwork you're doing here with the movement principles we covered in Chapter 8.

Stimulating the Vagus Nerve

The vagus nerve is like the main highway of your parasympathetic nervous system.[6] It runs from your brainstem down through your chest and abdomen, connecting to your heart, lungs, and digestive system. When it's functioning well, it helps keep your nervous system balanced.

When it's not, you get stuck in fight-or-flight mode.

Research has consistently shown that people with chronic pain conditions have reduced heart rate variability (HRV), a marker of vagal tone dysfunction.[7] This suggests that strengthening vagal tone through breathwork, meditation, or biofeedback may help regulate pain perception. Meta-analyses have shown that HRV biofeedback training can reduce stress, anxiety, and even pain by improving autonomic regulation.[8]

There are a few simple ways to stimulate the vagus nerve and encourage that parasympathetic response. Splash cold water on your face or hold an ice pack to your neck. The cold triggers a vagal response.[9] Hum or sing. The vibration activates vagal pathways.[10] It doesn't have to be good singing, just consistent. Gargle.

Same principle, as the physical stimulation activates the nerve.

These aren't miracle cures. But when done regularly, they can help shift your nervous system's baseline toward calm rather than alarm. And when your baseline shifts, everything else gets easier.

The Language of Movement: Integration and Practice

In Chapter 8, we covered movement as medicine in depth. How you can scale activity, pace yourself, and use graded exposure to retrain your nervous system. If you haven't implemented those principles yet, go back and start there. Movement is foundational.

But here's how it connects to everything else. Movement alone won't work if your nervous system is stuck in overdrive the rest of the day. And breath work alone won't build the strength and confidence that come from actually moving your body. These tools don't replace each other. They reinforce each other.

Your brain is constantly updating its body map based on input.[11] If you stop moving a certain way, the brain's representation of that movement becomes blurry or uncertain. But when you move gently and consistently within your limits, you're giving your brain clear, accurate information.

This is why physical therapy, yoga, tai chi, and even simple walking can be so effective.[12] Again, it's not about "fixing" damaged tissue, which often isn't the problem anyway. It's about retraining the brain. Every time you move without catastrophe, you're sending your nervous system a message: *This is safe. We can do this.* And eventually, your nervous system starts to believe it.

Qi gong, which we mentioned in the breath section, is one of the few practices that naturally combines breath, movement, and nervous system regulation without you having to think about it. The movements are slow, deliberate, and done within your current range of motion. No pushing, no forcing. Just moving your body in a way that signals safety while staying present with your breath.

If you're nervous about movement or if traditional exercise has failed you in the past, this is a good place to start. It doesn't feel like "exercise" in the conventional sense, which can make it less threatening to a nervous system that's learned to fear activity. You're just flowing through gentle movements, breathing deeply, staying present. And in doing so, you're teaching your brain that movement can be safe, even pleasant. Just remember to start slow here as well.

The key insight: *breath calms the system so movement feels safer. Movement builds confidence, so the system trusts breath work more. Sleep consolidates what you practiced during the day. And all of it works better when you're not isolated or constantly invalidated.*

That's integration. That's how these tools stack.

The Language of Nutrition: Reducing Unnecessary Stress

Let's be clear upfront. No diet is going to cure neuroplastic pain. If someone tells you that cutting out certain foods will fix your fibromyalgia, walk away. There are too many conflicting opinions, too many diet gurus promising miracles. And frankly, this isn't the book for nutritional prescriptions.

That said, what you eat does matter. Not because food causes your pain, but because chronic inflammation and blood sugar instability can amplify an already overactive nervous system.[13]

Think of it this way: your nervous system is already maxed out. It's dealing with distorted body maps, hyperactive threat detection, and a feedback loop that won't quit. Don't make it deal with preventable stressors on top of everything else.

Blood Sugar Stability

When your blood sugar spikes and crashes throughout the day, your body releases stress hormones to compensate.[14] Those stress hormones, cortisol and adrenaline, are the same ones that keep your nervous system in fight-or-flight mode.

Stable blood sugar equals a more stable nervous system.

You don't need a specific diet plan. You just need to notice patterns. Do you crash an hour after certain meals? Do you feel shaky or irritable mid-afternoon? Those are signs your blood sugar is unstable. Pay attention to what works for your body, not what works for someone else's Instagram feed.

Hydration

This one's almost too simple to mention, but dehydration is a sneaky pain amplifier.

When you're dehydrated, your blood volume drops, which means less oxygen and nutrients reach your tissues.[15] Your muscles get tighter. Your brain gets foggy. And your pain threshold drops.

If you're thirsty, you're already dehydrated. Aim for clear or pale yellow urine. If it's dark, drink more.

That's it. That's the nutrition section. I'm not going to tell you what to eat. You know your body better than I do. But recognize that if you're running on sugar crashes, caffeine spikes, and chronic dehydration, you're adding static to an already noisy system. Clean up what you can, and let your nervous system have one less thing to manage. And if you want to take it deeper, seek out a dietician or nutritionist who at least has a vague understanding of the conditions you are dealing with.

The Language of Connection: The Evolutionary Safety Signal

Chronic pain is isolating.

When you're in constant pain, you cancel plans. You stop going out. You withdraw from friends and family because it's easier than explaining for the hundredth time why you can't do something. And after a while, people stop asking.

The isolation makes everything worse. Not just emotionally, but physiologically.

Humans are social creatures. Our nervous systems are wired to regulate through connection.[16] When we feel seen, heard, and supported, our stress response calms. When we're isolated, the opposite happens. Our threat detection system ramps up.

This isn't just psychology. It's biology. In evolutionary terms, being cast out from the group was a death sentence.[17] Your nervous system still knows that. Isolation triggers the same threat response as physical danger.

The Hidden Stressors You're Not Counting

But isolation isn't the only relationship problem that keeps your nervous system stuck in high alert. Sometimes the problem isn't being alone. It's being with someone who drains you.

Stress isn't just about loud TVs, packed schedules, or too many notifications. It's also about relational load. The invisible weight of managing someone else's emotions, dysfunction, or instability.

Maybe it's a partner who can't hold down a job, cycles through substances, and functions more like another dependent than an equal. Perhaps it's a parent who requires constant emotional management. Maybe it's a friend who only shows up when they need something.

That constant vigilance doesn't feel like trauma. It doesn't look like PTSD. But it functions the same way. Your nervous system stays in protection mode because the threat never fully resolves. You can't relax because someone in your environment is fundamentally unsafe, even if they're not actively harmful.

Your brain is constantly scanning. Will they remember their responsibilities? Will they blow up the budget? Will you have to clean up another mess? That's not rest. That's not safety. That's chronic activation.

And your nervous system doesn't care if the stressor is "justified" or "understandable." It doesn't care if you love the person or if leaving feels impossible. It only knows whether you're safe or not. And if you're spending your days managing someone else's chaos, you're not safe.

I know we've covered this before, but it bears repeating, not just because it fits this chapter, but because it's often a significant catalyst in people's pain. It can become a blind spot; when the focus turns inward, they miss how much this factor contributes to what they're feeling. This isn't about blaming anyone. It's about recognizing that your relationships either feed your recovery or your pain. Sometimes, the most healing thing you can do is remove yourself from dynamics that keep your nervous system locked in threat mode.

The Validation You're Not Getting

One of the most damaging aspects of chronic pain is the constant invalidation. Doctors who dismiss your symptoms. Family members who imply you're exaggerating. Friends who say, "You don't look sick."

That invalidation doesn't just hurt your feelings. It activates your nervous system's threat response.[18] Your brain interprets invalidation as danger, because in our evolutionary past, social rejection meant you were vulnerable, alone, at risk.

Every time someone dismisses your pain, your nervous system gets the message: *You're not safe. No one believes you. You're on your own.* And that message amplifies everything.

Finding people who believe you, whether that's a support group, a therapist, or even an online community, can be a game-changer. Not because they fix your pain, but because they help your nervous system feel safer.

The Difficulty of Connection When You're Barely Functioning

Here's the cruel irony. When you most need connection, it's hardest to maintain.

You can't show up the way you used to. You can't commit to plans because you never know how you'll feel. You feel like a burden. You're exhausted from explaining yourself, defending yourself, and justifying your existence.

And so you withdraw. You isolate. And your nervous system interprets that isolation as further evidence that you're in danger.

Breaking that cycle doesn't mean forcing yourself to socialize when you feel terrible. It means finding small, manageable ways to maintain connection. A text to a friend. A phone call instead of an in-person visit. An online support group where you can show up in your pajamas.

You don't need a huge network. You just need a few people who get it. Who believe you. Who don't need you to explain or justify or prove anything.

Finding Your People (With Discernment)

Online support groups for fibromyalgia, EDS, or chronic pain can help. Reddit, Facebook, and dedicated forums. Therapists who specialize in chronic pain, especially those trained in CBT, ACT, or pain reprocessing therapy. Local support groups as well. To find them, check with hospitals or pain clinics in your area.

But here's something important to realize. Not all communities are helpful.

Some groups are full of people actively working toward healing. They share strategies, celebrate small wins, and support each other through setbacks. They acknowledge the struggle without drowning in it. These communities can be powerful.

Others, though, operate differently. They reinforce the idea that nothing works, that doctors are useless, and that hope is naive. The dominant narrative is: "We're all stuck, and anyone who gets better either wasn't really sick or got lucky." In these spaces, improvement is met with skepticism, and anyone who suggests a new approach is shut down.

Here's the thing: pain can become an identity. And when it does, letting go of it, even just a little, can feel like losing yourself. Some people aren't ready to heal, and that's their right. But if you're trying to move forward, surrounding yourself with people who are invested in staying stuck will make that nearly impossible.

So when you're looking for community, ask yourself:

Does this group encourage exploration, or does it shut down hope?

Healthy communities say, "That didn't work for me, but I'm glad you're trying."

Unhealthy ones say, "Don't bother. It won't work for you either."

Do people celebrate progress, or do they dismiss it?

Healthy communities cheer when someone has a good day.

Unhealthy ones respond with, "Just wait. It'll come back."

Is the focus on problem-solving, or venting without action?

Healthy communities share strategies, resources, and lessons learned.

Unhealthy ones loop endlessly on what's broken, without exploring what might help.

Do members support each other's agency, or reinforce helplessness?

Healthy communities say, "You know your body best. What feels right for you?"

Unhealthy ones say, "There's nothing you can do. You just have to accept it."

You're not looking for toxic positivity. You're not looking for people who pretend pain isn't real or who blame you for not healing fast enough. You're looking for people who hold space for both the struggle and the possibility of change.

If a community makes you feel more hopeless, more stuck, or more defined by your pain than you were before, it's okay to leave. In fact, it's imperative. You're not abandoning anyone. You're protecting your healing.

Connection signals safety to your nervous system in a way nothing else can. It tells your brain: *You're not alone. You're part of something. You're okay.*

And when your brain believes that, the volume starts to turn down.

The Language of Touch: Recalibrating Through Manual Therapy

Massage, physical therapy, chiropractic care, and acupuncture. These can all be valuable tools in your recovery toolkit. But they work for reasons you might not expect.

For years, manual therapy was thought to work by "fixing" tissues. Breaking up scar tissue, realigning bones, and releasing trigger points. But we now know that the real benefit comes from nervous system regulation.[19]

Research suggests that manual therapy may not work solely through mechanical "fixing" of tissues, but rather through neurophysiological mechanisms. Essentially, they recalibrate how the nervous system interprets input from the affected area.[20]

When a skilled therapist works on your body, several things happen. You receive focused, safe touch, which can calm an overactive nervous system. Studies have shown that massage can reduce pain, anxiety, and cortisol levels, suggesting it works by downregulating the stress response and calming the autonomic nervous system.[21] You're given permission to rest and receive care, which many chronic pain patients desperately need. The brain gets clear, non-threatening sensory input from the area being worked on, which can help update distorted body maps.[22] And trigger points and muscle tension often release, not because the tissue was damaged, but because the nervous system was holding that tension as a protective strategy.

Manual therapy works not by "fixing" your body, but by helping your nervous system feel safer.

What to Look For

If you're seeing a massage therapist or physical therapist, look for someone who understands pain science. Someone who talks about nervous system regulation, pacing, and graded exposure. Someone who doesn't promise to "fix" you but instead partners with you in your recovery.

Manual therapy can provide temporary relief from muscle tension and pain. It can help you connect with your body in a safe, supportive environment. It can serve as part of a broader recovery plan that includes sleep, movement, stress management, and nervous system regulation.

This isn't fringe thinking. Major medical guidelines now recommend massage and manual therapy as first-line treatments for conditions like chronic low back pain[23], and millions of people seek out these therapies specifically for pain relief.[24] The evidence base is solid. What's changed is our understanding of *why* it works.

But it can't cure your chronic pain on its own. It can't "fix" a structural problem that probably isn't the real issue anyway. And it won't work long-term unless you address the underlying nervous system dysfunction.

Think of manual therapy as one tool among many. Use it when it helps. But don't rely on it to do the work that only you can do.

Putting It All Together

None of these tools work in isolation. And none of them will work overnight.

But when you start stacking them, better sleep, stress management, gentle movement, stable nutrition, social connection, occasional bodywork, you create an environment where your nervous system can finally start to recalibrate.

Here's how they reinforce each other:

Sleep (Chapter 9) gives your nervous system the nightly reset it needs to consolidate what it learned during the day. Without it, nothing else sticks.

Movement (Chapter 8) teaches your brain that your body is safe and capable. It updates cortical maps and builds confidence.

Breath and regulation calm the system, so movement feels less threatening. They interrupt the stress loop that keeps pain amplified.

Nutrition reduces unnecessary stress via blood sugar crashes and dehydration, so your system has one less thing to manage.

Connection signals evolutionary safety. It tells your nervous system that you're not alone, that you're not cast out, that you're okay.

Touch provides focused, safe input that helps your brain update its maps and release protective tension.

Each one makes the others more effective. Movement works better when you're sleeping. Sleep improves when you're regulating stress during the day. Regulation is easier when you're connected. Connection is possible when you have the energy that comes from stable nutrition and restorative sleep.

This isn't about doing everything perfectly. It's about doing what you can, as consistently as you can, and trusting that small changes add up over time.

Your nervous system learned to amplify pain. It can also learn to turn it down. But it needs the right conditions to do so.

You're building those conditions. One breath, one step, one day at a time.

In the next chapter, we'll look at what happens when you start putting all of this into practice. What recovery actually looks like when you're living it, not just reading about it. The setbacks, the breakthroughs, the reality of learning to live in a body that's been at war with itself.

Because understanding the theory is one thing. Living it is another.

Reflection Prompt

Which of these recovery tools feels most accessible to you right now? Which feels most overwhelming? Start with what feels manageable, even if it's just one practice, and give yourself permission to build slowly from there. Recovery isn't about doing everything at once. It's about creating small, sustainable shifts that signal safety to your nervous system over time.

Endnotes

[1] Porges, S. W. (2011). *The Polyvagal Theory: Neurophysiological Foundations of Emotions, Attachment, Communication, and Self-regulation.* W.W. Norton & Company.

[2] Noble, D. J., & Hochman, S. (2019). Hypothesis: Oxygen and the autonomic nervous system—The oxygen–vagal theory. *Frontiers in Neuroscience, 13,* 454.

[3] Sapolsky, R. M. (2004). *Why Zebras Don't Get Ulcers* (3rd ed.). Holt Paperbacks.

[4] Zaccaro, A., Piarulli, A., Laurino, M., Garbella, E., Menicucci, D., Neri, B., & Gemignani, A. (2018). How breath-control can change your life: A systematic review on psycho-physiological correlates of slow breathing. *Frontiers in Human Neuroscience, 12,* 353.

[5] Ruscio, A. M., & Borkovec, T. D. (2004). Experience and appraisal of worry among high worriers with and without generalized anxiety disorder. *Behaviour Research and Therapy, 42*(12), 1469–1482.

[6] Porges, S. W. (2011). *The Polyvagal Theory: Neurophysiological Foundations of Emotions, Attachment,*

Communication, and Self-regulation. W.W. Norton & Company.

[7] Koenig, J., Jarczok, M. N., Ellis, R. J., Hillecke, T. K., & Thayer, J. F. (2014). Heart rate variability and experimentally induced pain in healthy adults: A systematic review. *European Journal of Pain*, 18(3), 301-314.

[8] Goessl, V. C., Curtiss, J. E., & Hofmann, S. G. (2017). The effect of heart rate variability biofeedback training on stress and anxiety: A meta-analysis. *Psychological Medicine*, 47(15), 2578-2586.

[9] Campbell, L. F. (1982). Diving Reflex in Man: Its Relation to Isometric and Dynamic Exercise. *Journal of Applied Physiology*, 52(1), 115-119.

[10] Vickhoff, B., et al. (2013). Music structure determines heart rate variability of singers. *Frontiers in Psychology*, 4, 334.

[11] Merzenich, M. M., & Jenkins, W. M. (1990). *Reorganization of cortical representations of the hand following alterations of skin inputs.* Brain Research, 525(2), 325–331.

[12] Hall, A. M., et al. (2016). The Effectiveness of Tai Chi for Chronic Musculoskeletal Pain Conditions: A

Systematic Review and Meta-analysis. *Arthritis & Rheumatology*, 69(9), 1876-1886.

[13] Hotamisligil, G. S. (2006). Inflammation and metabolic disorders. *Nature*, 444(7121), 860–867.

[14] Lassiter, D. G., et al. (2012). Counterregulatory responses to hypoglycemia. *Diabetes Care*, 35(6), 1380–1386.

[15] Popkin, B. M., et al. (2010). Water, hydration, and health. *Nutrition Reviews*, 68(8), 439-458.

[16] Coan, J. A., & Sbarra, D. A. (2015). Social Baseline Theory: The social regulation of risk and effort. *Current Opinion in Psychology*, 1, 87-91.

[17] Baumeister, R. F., & Leary, M. R. (1995). The need to belong: Desire for interpersonal attachments as a fundamental human motivation. *Psychological Bulletin*, 117(3), 497-529.

[18] Eisenberger, N. I., et al. (2003). Does rejection hurt? An fMRI study of social exclusion. *Science*, 302(5643), 290-292.

[19] Bialosky, J. E., et al. (2009). Placebo response to manual therapy: Something out of nothing? *Journal of Manual & Manipulative Therapy*, 17(1), 11-18.

[20] Bialosky, J. E., Bishop, M. D., Price, D. D., Robinson, M. E., & George, S. Z. (2009). The mechanisms of manual therapy in the treatment of musculoskeletal pain: A comprehensive model. *Manual Therapy*, 14(5), 531-538.

[21] Field, T. (2016). Massage therapy research review. *Complementary Therapies in Clinical Practice*, 24, 19-31.

[22] Moseley, G. L., & Flor, H. (2012). Targeting cortical representations in the treatment of chronic pain: A review. *Neurorehabilitation and Neural Repair*, 26(6), 646-652.

[23] Qaseem, A., et al. (2017). Noninvasive Treatments for Acute, Subacute, and Chronic Low Back Pain: A Clinical Practice Guideline From the American College of Physicians. *Annals of Internal Medicine*, 166(7), 514-530.

[24] National Center for Complementary and Integrative Health (NCCIH). (2021). Massage Therapy for Health Purposes: What You Need To Know. U.S. Department of Health and Human Services.

Chapter Eleven

Rebuilding Trust in Your Body

Trust doesn't work the way most people assume. Some people define it as the warm feeling of certainty, or the belief that everything will turn out fine. Others may even think it's the absence of doubt or fear. But trust is something quieter. And sometimes, it's harder won. It's the willingness to act despite uncertainty. It's showing up to the appointment when you're exhausted. It's trying the movement when you're scared. It's believing, just barely enough, that this time will be different.

For people living with chronic pain, trust is one of the first casualties. After years of failed treatments, dismissive doctors, and the relentless disappointment of hope deferred, the idea that anything could actually help feels dangerous. Hope becomes a liability. It's safer to expect nothing than to risk being let down again.

You've learned how pain works. You've started moving in ways that retrain your nervous system. By now, you hopefully understand the science behind maladaptive neuroplasticity and central sensitization. But knowing how the system works and trusting that your body can change are two different things. Knowledge doesn't automatically translate into belief. And without belief, even the best interventions feel like you're just going through the motions.

This chapter is about the psychological foundation that lies underneath everything else. It's about how you build it, even when your history screams that nothing will work. Because without trust, the techniques in earlier chapters remain theoretical. With it, they become transformative.

What Trust Actually Is (And Isn't)

Let's start by clearing up what trust isn't.

Trust is not confidence. Confidence says, "I know this will work." Trust says, "I don't know if this will work, but I'm willing to find out." Confidence requires certainty. Trust requires only willingness.[1]

Trust is not the absence of fear. You can be afraid and still trust. In fact, that's usually how it works. The person with chronic pain who tries a new movement despite fearing a flare. Or the patient who walks into another clinic after a dozen failures. These aren't people without fear; they're people acting in the presence of fear. That's trust.

Trust is also not permanent. It's not something you achieve once and keep forever. It's a practice, rebuilt daily, sometimes multiple times a day. It fluctuates, and that's normal.

So, what is trust actually? When discussing the concepts here, it's best to define trust as **the accumulated evidence that contradicts your worst predictions.**

You expected disaster, and it didn't happen. You thought the flare would last weeks, and it lasted three days. You anticipated crushing pain after a walk, and instead, you felt tired but manageable. These small contradictions stack up over time, slowly rewriting the story your nervous system has been telling itself.[2]

The brain is a prediction machine. It's constantly generating expectations based on experience. When you've been hurt repeatedly, regardless of the type, the brain learns to predict harm. It becomes efficient at assuming the worst because, historically, that's been accurate.[3] Trust begins when new data challenges those predictions. Not once. Not twice. But repeatedly and consistently. And most of all, undeniably.

Reflection Prompt

Think about a time when you expected the worst and it didn't happen. How did your body respond? Did you notice that moment, or did your mind immediately dismiss it as a fluke?

The Three Dimensions of Trust

Trust doesn't build in one direction; rather, it accumulates across three interconnected dimensions. These can be labeled as physical, emotional, and behavioral. Each reinforces the others, creating a feedback loop that either strengthens or undermines the whole system.

Physical Trust: Evidence from the Body

Physical trust comes from the body's direct experience of safety. It's built through movement that doesn't cause disaster, as well as through activities that once seemed impossible, becoming possible again. It can even be built through flares that resolve faster than expected.

Chapter 8 taught us that graded movement exposure teaches the nervous system that motion is safe. But it's not just the mechanical dimension that matters here;

the psychological one matters as well. It's not just that the tissue can handle the load, it's that *YOU believe it can*. And that belief doesn't come from pep talks. It comes from repeated, lived experience.[4]

Consider someone who's avoided stairs for two years. This could be because the last time they tried, their knee swelled for a week. So now, they start with a single step, twice a day, holding the rail. Nothing catastrophic happens. A week later, they try two steps. Still fine. Three weeks in, they're doing a full flight without bracing for impact. The movement capacity was always there, waiting to be accessed. What changed wasn't the knee. It was the belief that the knee could be trusted.

That's physical trust. Not "my body is invincible," but "my body is more capable than I've been giving it credit for."

Emotional Trust: Reframing Interpretation

Emotional trust is cognitive. It's the ability to reinterpret sensations in ways that don't spiral into catastrophe.

A twinge doesn't automatically mean that there is an injury. Soreness after activity doesn't mean you've destroyed progress. And a flare doesn't mean you're back to square one. These reframes don't happen because you talk yourself into positivity. They happen because you have evidence.[5]

The Pain Catastrophizing Scale measures how people interpret pain sensations: magnification (seeing pain as worse than it is), rumination (obsessing over it), and helplessness (believing nothing can be done).[6] High catastrophizing isn't a character flaw. It's a learned response. When pain has been unpredictable, overwhelming, and unresponsive to treatment, catastrophizing makes sense. Your brain is trying to protect you. But it's doing so by assuming the worst.

Emotional trust is the slow unlearning of that pattern. Think of it as tracking data that contradicts catastrophic predictions. "I thought this flare would ruin my week, but I was functional again in two days." "I expected this activity to set me back, but I recovered faster than last time." It's not blind optimism, it's a correct interpretation of evidence.

This dimension loops back into physical trust. When you expect movement to hurt, you brace, amplifying the signal. But when you expect movement to be manageable, you relax, and the signal stays quieter.[7] The mind doesn't just observe the body. It shapes what the body experiences.

Behavioral Trust: Showing Up Anyway

Behavioral trust is action. It's walking into the clinic even when you're skeptical. It's trying the exercise even when you doubt it will help. Or something as simple as journaling your wins, even when they feel insignificant.

This is where trust becomes tangible. You can think positive thoughts all day, but if you're not acting on them, the nervous system doesn't update. Behavior is the language the brain understands best.[8]

Behavioral trust often comes last. You don't believe it will work, so you show up with low expectations. But you show up. And that act of showing up time after time becomes its own form of evidence. "I didn't think this would help, but I kept coming back. And now I'm noticing changes."

The three dimensions feed each other. Physical wins create emotional reframes, and emotional reframes make behavioral follow-through easier. And behavioral follow-through generates more physical wins. The loop can work for you just as powerfully as it once worked against you.

How Trust Builds Over Time

Trust doesn't appear overnight. It accumulates in stages, each one building on the last.

Early Stage: Skepticism to Curiosity

At first, trust isn't about belief. It's about curiosity.

Most people with chronic pain start treatment after years of failed attempts. The first emotion isn't hope. It's wariness. "This probably won't work either." That's not pessimism. That's self-preservation. After trying "everything" and having nothing work, walking into yet another clinic requires a particular kind of courage. And when something finally does start working, the first response isn't relief. It's disbelief.[9]

"This is probably just a fluke."

"I'm sure it won't last."

"It's just a good week."

These dismissals aren't about being difficult. They're about protecting yourself from another round of disappointment. Because if you believe it's working and then it stops, you're not sure you can survive that emotional collapse again.

The shift from skepticism to curiosity is subtle but significant. Skepticism says, "This won't work." Curiosity says, "I wonder if this might work." That small opening, from closed to tentatively open, is where everything begins.

Often, understanding the mechanism helps. When someone learns that their pain pattern isn't random but follows the logic of cortical remapping, it makes sense even when it feels senseless. It's at this point that something shifts. The pain isn't proof of being broken. It's proof of a system that learned too well. And what's learned can be unlearned.[10]

You can see the shift in body language. Early on, patients sit with arms crossed and eyes down. They likely even give one-word answers. But after a few weeks, they're leaning forward, asking questions, reporting small wins. "I carried the groceries without a flare." "I slept through the night." "I didn't think about my pain for an entire afternoon." These aren't monumental victories, but they're undeniable. And undeniable is what trust needs to grow.

Middle Stage: Accumulating Evidence

This is where trust gets real work done. You've had enough small wins that dismissing them as flukes becomes harder. The pattern is starting to show itself.

A flare happens again. But instead of lasting two weeks, it resolves in four days. You test a movement you've been avoiding, and it's still uncomfortable. But now it's at least manageable. Or a more subtle observation might be that you wake up one morning and realize you didn't check your pain level first thing because it just wasn't the loudest signal in your awareness.

The nervous system is updating its predictions. Movement that once triggered alarm bells now registers as neutral. Activities that felt dangerous now feel possible. The map is being redrawn, one experience at a time.[11]

But this stage is also where trust gets tested. Because progress isn't linear, and setbacks still happen.

A bad flare hits. You may have pushed too hard, or it may have come out of nowhere. Suddenly, all the progress feels fragile. The catastrophic thoughts rush back. "I knew this wouldn't last. I'm back to square one."

Here's where trust matters most. Do you interpret the flare as proof of failure? Or do you interpret it as temporary data? Do you spiral into helplessness? Or do you contextualize it?

Trust at this stage means recognizing that a bad week isn't a bad life. It means having enough accumulated evidence that one setback doesn't erase everything. It means adjusting instead of collapsing.[12]

Someone with robust middle-stage trust might think: "This flare sucks. But the last three resolved faster than they used to. I know what to do. I'll scale back, rest, and check in with my provider if it doesn't improve in a few days." That's not toxic positivity. That's an accurate risk assessment based on evidence.

Late Stage: Trust Becomes Quiet

Six months in, you're not thinking about pain as much. It's background noise, not the main event. You have more bandwidth for other things. You make plans without calculating whether your body can handle them.

A year in, you've weathered multiple flares and recovered from all of them. The pattern is undeniable.

You know what to do when symptoms spike. You don't panic. You adjust.

Long-term, trust becomes so ingrained that you stop noticing it. You don't announce it. You don't need to prove it to yourself anymore. You just live it.

The most profound sign of trust isn't confidence. It's forgetting to be afraid. You reach for something, stand up from a chair, bend down to pick something up, and it's only afterward that you realize you didn't brace. You didn't hold your breath. You didn't mentally calculate the risk. You just moved.[13]

That's when you know the nervous system has truly updated. The prediction has changed from "this will hurt" to "this is fine."

But even at this stage, trust doesn't mean you never doubt. It means you move forward anyway. You don't need perfect trust. You just need enough.

When Trust Breaks: Navigating Setbacks

Trust isn't fragile. But it's not invincible either. Major flares can crack the foundation that you've been building. Failed treatments or dismissive interactions can widen those cracks. How you respond to them determines whether trust collapses or adapts.

The Anatomy of a Trust-Breaking Event

Let's say you've been doing well for three months. Pain levels have dropped. You've been moving more, sleeping better, and feeling hopeful. Then you try something new. Maybe you increased your walking distance, maybe you attended a social event that required more energy than usual, and you crash. Hard.

The pain is back at levels you haven't experienced in weeks. The fatigue is crushing. And the thought loop starts immediately: "I knew this wouldn't last. I'm broken. Nothing actually works."

This moment is critical. If you interpret the flare as proof that all progress was illusory, trust will collapse. But if you interpret it as a temporary strain on a system that's still recalibrating, your trust continues to adapt.

The difference comes down to context. A flare isn't random; it's data. What triggered it? Was it a massive overreach, or a reasonable progression that happened to hit a sensitive threshold? How does this flare compare to past flares in intensity and duration? What do you know now that you didn't know three months ago?

Trust doesn't mean nothing ever goes wrong. It means you can contextualize what goes wrong rather than catastrophize it.[14]

Rebuilding After a Breach

If a major setback has shaken your trust, rebuilding starts small. You don't need to believe the whole system works again. You just need to believe one small thing might work.

That could be a single session with a trusted provider. It could be one graded movement that has worked before. It could be revisiting your tracking data to remind yourself of progress that's already happened.

The goal is to create enough safety that you are willing to try again. It is not to erase doubt. And then you let the evidence pile up, one small contradictory data point at a time.

Trust Across Conditions

Trust varies for each individual, influenced by their unique history and experiences. The timeline and required evidence can vary significantly depending on personal circumstances. Many individuals have distinct fears regarding elements that may exacerbate their pain.

For someone with fibromyalgia, physical trust might mean learning that not every sensation is a warning sign. Emotional trust might mean distinguishing between "hurt" and "harm." Behavioral trust might mean showing up to movement practice even when you're tired, because you know fatigue doesn't equal danger.

For someone with EDS, physical trust might mean believing that controlled movement can strengthen stability rather than cause injury. Emotional trust might mean reframing joint instability as something to manage rather than something that defines you. Behavioral trust might mean pacing without guilt.

For someone with CRPS, physical trust might start with desensitization, simply touching the affected limb without spiraling into panic. Emotional trust might mean separating the sensation from the catastrophic meaning you've assigned to it. Behavioral trust might mean engaging with graded motor imagery even when it feels pointless.

The specifics differ, but the principles remain the same. Trust is built on evidence and sustained by consistency.

Most of all, it's deepened through successfully navigating setbacks.

Practical Tools for Tracking Trust

Trust is easier to build when you can see it accumulating. These tools help make the invisible visible.

The Win Log

Every day, write down one thing that went better than expected. It doesn't have to be big. You may have been able to stand for 10 minutes without pain, and/or get 6 hours of quality sleep. You may have even noticed when you caught a catastrophic thought, but were able to reframe it this time. Over time, this log becomes undeniable evidence that things are changing.[15]

The Flare Journal

When a flare hits, track: What triggered it (if known)? How intense was it (0-10 scale)? How long did it last? What helped? How does it compare to previous flares? This turns flares from proof of failure into data points that inform your approach.

The Fear Ladder

List activities you've been avoiding, ranked from least to most intimidating. Start with the easiest one. When you complete it without catastrophe, move to the next. This creates a visible progression of trust-building.

The Expectation vs. Reality Check

Before trying something new, write down what you expect to happen. Afterward, write down what actually happened. Over time, you'll see the gap between catastrophic predictions and manageable reality. That gap is where trust grows.

Trust as Daily Practice

Trust isn't a destination. It's a practice you return to daily, sometimes multiple times a day.

Some days, trust feels solid. You move through the world with ease, barely thinking about pain. Other days, trust feels shaky. A bad night of sleep, a minor flare, a dismissive comment from someone who doesn't understand. Any of these can rattle the foundation.

On those shaky days, trust isn't about feeling certain. It's about remembering what you know. It's pulling out your win log and reading through it. It's reminding yourself that the last flare resolved. It's choosing to show up to one small practice even when you don't feel like it.

Trust compounds. Each small act reinforces the next. Each successfully managed flare deepens the foundation. Each moment you choose to act despite doubt strengthens the pathway.[16]

You don't need to have perfect trust to move forward. You just need enough to try one more session. Enough to question one more catastrophic thought. Enough to believe that your body isn't the enemy.

Progress isn't linear. Trust isn't either. But both accumulate over time. And accumulation, not perfection, is what creates lasting change.

In the next chapter, we'll explore what it means to carry this trust into a world that doesn't always understand chronic pain. And how to protect what you've built when the people around you don't reinforce it.

Endnotes

[1] Harrison, F., & McLaughlin, K. A. (2019). Cognitive mechanisms of psychotherapy: Prediction, learning, and trust in the therapeutic process. *Current Opinion in Psychology*, 30, 44–49.

[2] Cormier, S., Lavigne, G. L., Choinière, M., & Rainville, P. (2016). Expectations predict chronic pain treatment outcomes. *Pain*, 157(2), 329–338.

[3] Büchel, C., Geuter, S., Sprenger, C., & Eippert, F. (2014). Placebo analgesia: A predictive coding perspective. *Neuron*, 81(6), 1223–1239.

[4] Vlaeyen, J. W., & Linton, S. J. (2012). Fear-avoidance model of chronic musculoskeletal pain: 12 years on. *Pain*, 153(6), 1144–1147.

[5] Vlaeyen, J. W., & Linton, S. J. (2012). Fear-avoidance model of chronic musculoskeletal pain: 12 years on. *Pain*, 153(6), 1144–1147.

[6] Sullivan, M. J., Bishop, S. R., & Pivik, J. (1995). The Pain Catastrophizing Scale: Development and validation. *Psychological Assessment*, 7(4), 524–532.

[7] Eccleston, C., & Crombez, G. (2007). Worry and chronic pain: A misdirected problem solving model. *Pain*, 132(3), 233–236.

[8] Moseley, G. L., & Butler, D. S. (2015). Fifteen years of explaining pain: The past, present, and future. *Journal of Pain*, 16(9), 807–813.

[9] West, C., Stewart, L., Foster, K., & Usher, K. (2012). The meaning of chronic pain: A qualitative meta-synthesis. International Journal of Nursing Studies, 49(6), 698–710.

[10] Butler, D. S., & Moseley, G. L. (2013). *Explain Pain* (2nd ed.). Noigroup Publications.

[11] Flor, H. (2012). New developments in the understanding and management of persistent pain. *Current Opinion in Psychiatry*, 25(2), 109–113.

[12] Pincus, T., & McCracken, L. M. (2013). Psychological factors and treatment opportunities in low back pain. *Best Practice & Research Clinical Rheumatology*, 27(5), 625–635.

[13] Myers, K. M., & Davis, M. (2007). Mechanisms of fear extinction. *Neuron*, 56(5), 829–844.

[14] Pincus, T., & McCracken, L. M. (2013). Psychological factors and treatment opportunities in low back pain. *Best Practice & Research Clinical Rheumatology*, 27(5), 625–635.

[15] Hughes, L. S., Clark, J., Colclough, J. A., Dale, E., & McMillan, D. (2017). Acceptance and Commitment Therapy (ACT) for chronic pain: A systematic review and meta-analyses. *The Clinical Journal of Pain*, 33(6), 552–568.

[16] McCracken, L. M., & Vowles, K. E. (2014). Acceptance and Commitment Therapy and mindfulness for chronic pain: Model, process, and progress. *American Psychologist*, 69(2), 178–187.

Chapter Twelve

Living in a World That Does Not Understand

In Chapter 11, we explored how trust is rebuilt internally through accumulated evidence. We discussed small wins, such as reframed experiences, and the slow realization that your body can adapt. In this chapter, we'll talk about carrying that trust into a world that won't always reinforce it. And, how to protect what you've built when the people around you don't understand.

Because here's the truth. Not everyone will get it. Some won't even try. And living with chronic pain in a world built for people without it requires a different kind of navigation. This chapter is about that navigation. About how you can translate your experience without exhausting yourself. How to set boundaries without guilt. And how to protect your identity when the world keeps telling you that you're lazy, weak, or imagining things.

This isn't about becoming a better advocate or educator. It's about surviving, and sometimes, maybe even thriving, in spaces that weren't designed with you in mind.

The Cost No One Sees

Chronic pain is invisible, and invisibility comes with a cost.

When someone breaks their leg, the cast tells the story. People hold doors. They offer to carry things. They don't question why you're moving slowly or why you can't make it to dinner. The injury is visible, so the accommodations feel justified. No one asks you to prove it.

But chronic pain doesn't come with a cast. You look fine. You've learned to smile through it, to function through it, to show up even when every cell in your body is screaming. And because people can't see it, they assume it's not that bad. Or worse, they think it's not real.

You've heard the comments. "You don't look sick." "I get tired too." "Have you tried yoga?" These aren't just frustrating. They're isolating. Because what they're really saying is: I don't believe you. Or at least, I don't believe it's as bad as you say it is.

And over time, that isolation compounds. You stop mentioning the pain because you're tired of defending it. You cancel plans, and people stop inviting you. You pull back from relationships that require too much explaining, and the world around you shrinks. Not because you want it to, but because navigating misunderstanding takes energy you don't have.[1]

The cost of invisibility isn't just social. It's neurological. Research shows that social rejection activates the same brain regions as physical pain: the anterior cingulate cortex and the insula.[2] Your nervous system doesn't distinguish between being dismissed by a doctor and being dismissed by a friend. Both are registered as threats. Both reinforce the vigilance you're trying to calm. And both make it harder to hold onto the trust you've been rebuilding.

This is the backdrop against which you're trying to heal. You're not just managing pain. You're managing a world that doesn't see it, doesn't understand it, and often doesn't believe it. And that requires a level of self-protection that goes beyond physical pacing. It requires emotional and relational pacing, too.

Reflection Prompt

When was the last time you felt truly seen and believed about your pain? What made that moment different?

Why Dismissal Matters

Dismissal isn't neutral. It's not just annoying or inconvenient. It has measurable effects on pain outcomes, nervous system regulation, and your ability to trust the healing process.[3]

Let's break down the types of dismissal you're likely encountering and why each one matters.

Medical Dismissal

This is the doctor who tells you your test results are normal, so there's nothing wrong. The specialist who suggests it's "just stress" or "probably anxiety." The physical therapist who doesn't believe hypermobility could cause this much pain. The provider who implies you're drug-seeking when you ask for help managing symptoms.

Medical dismissal doesn't just waste time; it also harms patients. It teaches your nervous system that help isn't coming. And when the brain believes no external support is available, it doubles down on internal threat signals. The pain amplifies. The hypervigilance increases. The very system you're trying to calm gets louder.[4]

Research on therapeutic alliance, the trust and collaboration between patient and provider, shows that dismissal actively worsens pain outcomes. Patients who feel invalidated by their providers report higher pain intensity, greater disability, and poorer treatment adherence.[5] It's not that they're being difficult. It's that their nervous system is responding to the lack of safety in the therapeutic relationship.

Let's be clear about something before we go further. We have briefly mentioned this in the introduction and Chapter 7. Still, it is crucial to explore it in greater depth in this chapter, as it is such an important aspect to understand when discussing dismissal. When we talk in this book about doctors dismissing patients or physical therapists not understanding what to do, I'm not painting them as villains. Yes, there are bad actors, doctors who don't listen and write you off. PTs who don't care or don't get it. But these are the exception, not the rule. The vast majority of healthcare providers actually do give a damn.

That doctor who tells you nothing's wrong? He's run the tests and found nothing. In his mind, there's nothing to treat, and he believes his confidence has to outweigh your doubt. This isn't to make you feel crazy; it's an attempt to give you peace of mind and help you trust in his expertise. The problem is, it doesn't make the pain go away, which is why it usually lands as a dismissal.

Or take the physical therapist hammering you with their protocol. They have a timeline. We all know that the second you start seeing results, insurance stops paying for treatment. This leaves physical therapists trying to get as much done as they can in the short window insurance allows them to work on you. In many cases, the treatment protocols are actually dictated by the insurance companies, by what they'll pay for and what they won't. It's not that they're trying to flare you up or don't believe you when you say that work hurts. It's that they have to try and get results before the well runs dry and sessions are forced to halt.

This is why understanding this framework is so essential for better communication. When your doctor wants to assure you that you're okay because the test results are normal, you must both be able to understand that you might be looking in the wrong place. You need to explain the need for someone or something to address central sensitization, not structural or mechanical damage. The same goes for physical therapy. It's vital to understand where they're coming from, as well as what you actually need, so you can communicate that you may need something to help the nervous system adapt and not feel threatened. Something you could build upon even after the sessions stop. And then, when insurance covers expenses again, you could follow their baseline protocol and progress from there to avoid flare-ups the next time.

After all of this, however, it's important to know that if the medical system has dismissed you, it's not your fault. And it's not proof that your pain is imaginary. It's proof that the system doesn't have adequate frameworks for understanding complex pain. That's a failure of the system, not of you.

Social Dismissal

This is the friend who says, "But you were fine yesterday." The family member who tells you to "just push through it." The partner who sighs when you can't make it to another event. The coworker who makes passive-aggressive comments about your "flexibility" with deadlines.

Social dismissal cuts deeper because it comes from people who are supposed to care about you. And it compounds the isolation. When the people closest to you don't believe or understand, where do you go?

The neurological impact is real. Social pain from exclusion, rejection, and/or dismissal activates the same neural circuits as physical pain.[6] Your brain doesn't distinguish between being physically hurt and being socially excluded. Both are processed as threats to survival. And both keep the nervous system on high alert, making pain more difficult to manage.

This doesn't mean you need everyone in your life to understand. But it does mean you need at least a few people who do. And if those people don't exist yet, finding them becomes part of the work.

Workplace Dismissal

This is the manager who questions your need for accommodations. The HR department that treats your condition like an inconvenience. The colleagues who make comments about "special treatment" or joke about your sick days. The unspoken pressure to prove you're still productive, still valuable, still worth keeping around.

Workplace dismissal is particularly insidious because it's tied to financial security. You can't just walk away. You need the job. So you push through, overfunction, hide the pain, and pay for it later with crashes that no one sees.

The Americans with Disabilities Act (ADA) provides protections for people with chronic pain. However, enforcement is inconsistent, as many employers are either ignorant of the law or even openly hostile to accommodation requests.[7] Navigating this landscape requires documentation, persistence, and often legal knowledge that feels overwhelming when you're already exhausted.

You don't owe your employer perfect health. You don't owe them overperformance to justify your existence. But living in a system that implies otherwise takes a psychological toll that's easy to underestimate.

Translation, Not Persuasion

The truth is simple. You don't need to convince anyone. You don't need to defend your experience. You don't need to turn every interaction into an educational opportunity about chronic pain.

What you do need is a way to communicate that protects your energy, sets expectations, and maintains boundaries, all without burning yourself out in the process.

This is where translation comes in. Not persuasion. Not justification. Just clear, simple communication that says enough without saying too much.

The Elevator Pitch

An elevator pitch is a 30-second explanation that provides essential information without inviting debate. It's not comprehensive. It's not scientifically detailed. It's just enough to set the context so you can move forward.

Here's an example:

"I have a chronic pain condition that affects my nervous system. Some days are better than others. But I've learned to pace myself to avoid flare-ups. I appreciate your understanding."

That's all you need to say. No need to discuss maladaptive neuroplasticity or cortical remapping. No justification for why the pain is real. Just a clear boundary that reinforces that this is your reality, and you're managing it.

You can adapt this for different contexts.

To a friend: "I'm dealing with an unpredictable chronic pain condition. I want to hang out, but I might need to cancel at the last minute if I'm flaring. It's not personal, it's just how my body works right now."

To an employer: "I have a medical condition that requires some flexibility in my schedule. I'm fully capable of doing my job. But I may need occasional accommodations, like adjusting my hours or working from home during flare-ups."

To a family member: "I know it's hard to understand because you can't see it. I'm managing a condition that causes significant pain and fatigue. I'm doing everything I can to get better, and I need your support, not your advice."

The goal isn't to make them understand everything. It's to give them enough information to adjust their expectations.

When to Educate

Some people are genuinely curious. They want to understand. They ask good questions. They listen without interrupting. For these people, a deeper explanation might be worth your energy.

But even then, gauge your capacity. Educating others about chronic pain is labor. Emotionally and cognitively. And you don't owe it to anyone just because they're interested.

If you do choose to educate, keep it concrete

"My nervous system has learned to amplify pain signals even when there's no injury. It's like an alarm system that won't turn off. I'm retraining it through movement. I'm also focusing on improving my sleep and even practicing nervous system regulation techniques. But it takes time."

That gives them the framework without requiring a neuroscience lecture. If they want more, they can ask. If they don't, you've said enough.

When to Boundary Instead

Most people don't need the full explanation. They need a boundary.

"I appreciate your concern, but I'm working with my care team on this."

"I'm not looking for advice right now, but thank you."

"I'd rather not talk about my health. How's your week been?"

These aren't rude. They're clear. And clarity is kindness, to them and to you.

If someone pushes back, that's information. It tells you they're more interested in being right than in respecting your boundary. And that tells you how much energy they're worth.

Reflection Prompt

Think of someone in your life who doesn't understand your condition. What would a clear, simple translation sound like for them?

Boundary Architecture

Boundaries aren't about building walls. They're about deciding what comes in, and more importantly, what stays out. They're about protecting your energy, your trust that you've worked to build, and your nervous system from inputs that undermine your healing.

Not all boundaries look the same. Some are soft, gentle redirections that preserve the relationship. Some are hard, firm limits that protect you from harm. Knowing which to use, and when, is part of the skill of living well with chronic pain.

Soft Boundaries: Redirecting Without Rupture

Soft boundaries are for people who mean well but don't fully understand. They're not trying to hurt you. They're just operating from a different framework. These boundaries gently steer the conversation without creating conflict.

Examples:

When someone offers unsolicited advice

"I appreciate that you're trying to help. Right now, I'm following a plan with my providers, and I'm not looking to add anything new."

When someone questions your limits

"I know it's hard to understand from the outside. I've learned what my body can handle, and I'm sticking to that."

When someone compares their experience to yours

"I hear you, everyone's tired sometimes. What I'm dealing with is a bit different, but I'm managing it."

Soft boundaries preserve the relationship while making it clear that the topic isn't open for debate. They're your first line of defense for people who care about you but need gentle redirection.

Hard Boundaries: Protecting What Matters

Hard boundaries are for people who repeatedly overstep or dismiss you. Some may even try to undermine you. These aren't negotiations. They're firm limits that protect your well-being.

Examples:

When someone refuses to respect your limits

"I've explained my situation. I'm not going to keep defending it. If you can't respect that, we'll need to end this conversation."

When someone uses your pain against you

"That's not okay. I'm not going to discuss this with you anymore."

When someone demands more than you can give

"I understand that's frustrating for you, but I can't do that right now. This is my limit."

Hard boundaries often feel uncomfortable because we're taught that saying no is unkind. But protecting yourself from harm isn't unkind. It's necessary.

When to Walk Away

Some relationships can't adapt, and that's not your failure. It's just the reality of incompatibility.

If someone in your life refuses to respect your boundaries by repeatedly dismissing your experience or actively undermining your progress, you have permission to step back.

This doesn't mean cutting people off at the first sign of misunderstanding. It means recognizing when chronic invalidation is doing more harm than the relationship is worth. Some people will never understand. Some won't even try. And some will use your pain as a weapon, either to control you, to diminish you, or to center their own discomfort.

You don't owe those people access to your healing. You don't owe them explanations, second chances, or emotional labor. What you owe yourself is protection.[8]

Walking away isn't failure. Its boundaries in their most honest form.

What About Online Spaces?

Online chronic pain communities can be lifelines. They can also be traps.

The good ones offer validation, shared knowledge, and a sense of belonging that's hard to find elsewhere. But some communities become echo chambers of hopelessness, where improvement is dismissed as luck or betrayal, where trying new things is seen as naive, and where the shared identity revolves around suffering rather than adaptation.

If a community makes you feel more hopeless, more stuck, or more afraid to try anything new, it's time to step back. You needed that space when you needed it. But if it's reinforcing the very patterns you're trying to shift, it's no longer serving you.

You can leave quietly. You don't owe anyone an explanation. And you can always come back later if you want to. But right now, your job is to protect the part of you that still believes things can change.

Protecting Your Energy

Pacing doesn't only apply to movement. It applies to people, places, and information. Social and sensory overload can push your nervous system back into high alert, making it harder to maintain the trust you've built.[9]

Managing your social energy isn't about avoiding life. It's about engaging with life in a way that doesn't cost you days of recovery.

Limit information overload:

Doomscrolling at night, constant news updates, endless health research, all of these tax your nervous system. Set boundaries around when and how much information you consume. Your brain needs rest from input, not just activity.

Social Pacing Strategies

Simplify contact when needed

Commit to shorter visits or phone calls instead of longer ones, like a 30-minute coffee instead of a three-hour dinner. Or, a text check-in instead of a video call. You're not withdrawing. You're dosing your social energy in ways your nervous system can handle.

Choose environments wisely

Overstimulating environments, such as loud restaurants and crowded events, can drain your reserves more quickly. When possible, suggest quieter alternatives. A walk in the park instead of a bar, or A small gathering instead of a large party. Your environment matters.

Build in recovery breaks

If you're attending an event, plan your exit strategy. Step outside for five minutes. Find a quiet corner to breathe. Sit in your car before heading home. These micro-recoveries prevent the complete crash later.

Imagine this scenario. You've been invited to your cousin's birthday party. You want to go, but you already know what to expect. Loud music, and overlapping conversations that can create an influx of stimulus to your nervous system. And to throw gas on the fire, a crowd of people who don't understand why you "look fine" but can't stay for hours.

Here's how you might pace it.

Before the event

Decide in advance that you'll stay for ninety minutes, not the full three hours. Let one trusted person know you might be leaving early, so you don't have to explain to everyone. Eat a small meal beforehand so you're not reliant on party food that might trigger symptoms.

During the event

Arrive after the initial rush when energy is slightly calmer. Position yourself near an exit or a quieter corner. Take a break halfway through, step outside, sit in your car, or find a bathroom where you can close the door and breathe for five minutes. If someone asks why you're leaving early, use a soft boundary: "I had a great time, but I need to head out."

After the event

Build in recovery time. Don't schedule anything demanding for the next day. If you flare, remind yourself that it's not failure, it's your nervous system processing a higher-than-usual sensory load. Track what worked and what didn't so you can adjust next time.

This kind of planning isn't overthinking. It's intelligent pacing. And it's what allows you to participate in life without sacrificing days of function afterward.

Another Example could look like this. Let's say your job requires you to attend a three-day conference. There's no opting out. The days are long, the environment is overstimulating, and you know you'll pay for it.

Here's how you protect yourself.

Before

Book a hotel room even if you live locally. You need a space to retreat to between sessions. Pack earplugs, an eye mask, and anything else that helps you regulate.

Communicate with your supervisor ahead of time: "I'll be attending the key sessions, but I may need to step out periodically to manage my energy."

During

Skip the optional networking events. Attend the sessions that matter most and give yourself permission to miss the rest. Use breaks to lie down in your hotel room, not to socialize. Bring snacks, so you're not forced to rely on conference food.

After

Request the day after the conference off, or at a minimum, a reduced schedule. Don't try to jump back into normal work immediately. Give your system time to recover.

You're not being difficult. You're being strategic. And strategic is what allows you to keep showing up.

Reflection Prompt

What's one social situation you've been avoiding because you don't know how to pace it? How might you approach it differently?

Identity Beyond Pain

The most significant danger of living in a world that doesn't understand isn't the dismissal itself. It's internalizing it and starting to believe the lies that you're lazy, weak, crazy, or broken.

Here's where the book comes full circle. You've seen the science. You have the framework. You understand what's happening in your nervous system. Other people's confusion doesn't define your reality. And your identity isn't built on other people's misunderstanding. It's built on the work you're doing: scaling, pacing, recalibrating, rebuilding trust. Every small win is a brick in your foundation. Every flare that's shorter than the last. Every task you reclaim, and every night of better sleep, these are the truths you build your identity on.

Carrying It Forward

You've learned the science. You've rebuilt trust internally. You understand how your nervous system works and what it needs to recalibrate. Now you're carrying that knowledge into a world that doesn't always reinforce it.

This is ongoing work, not a destination. Some days, protecting your trust will feel effortless. Other days, it will feel like swimming against the current. Both are normal.

The goal isn't to make everyone understand. It's to create enough space, physical, emotional, relational, for your healing to continue even when the world doesn't validate it.

You've built the foundation. Now you're learning to live on it. And that's not easy, but it's possible. Because you're not broken. You're adaptable. And adaptation means there's always a way forward, even when the path isn't clear.

In the next chapter, we'll bring it all together. Movement, sleep, recalibration, trust, protection, all of it. And we will give you a framework for writing your own map forward. Because this book isn't the end. It's the beginning.

Endnotes

¹ Sturgeon, J. A., & Zautra, A. J. (2016). Social pain and physical pain: Shared paths to resilience. *Pain Management*, 6(1), 63–74.

² Eisenberger, N. I., Lieberman, M. D., & Williams, K. D. (2003). Does rejection hurt? An fMRI study of social exclusion. *Science*, 302(5643), 290–292.

³ Eisenberger, N. I. (2012). Broken hearts and broken bones: A neural perspective on the similarities between social and physical pain. *Current Directions in Psychological Science*, 21(1), 42–47.

⁴ Cano, A., & Williams, A. C. (2010). Social interaction in pain: Reinforcing pain behaviors or building intimacy? *Pain*, 149(1), 9–11.

⁵ Fuentes, J., et al. (2014). Enhanced therapeutic alliance modulates pain intensity and muscle pain sensitivity in patients with chronic low back pain: An experimental controlled study. *Physical Therapy*, 94(4), 477–489.

⁶ Eisenberger, N. I., & Cole, S. W. (2012). Social neuroscience and health: Neurophysiological

mechanisms linking social ties with physical health. *Nature Neuroscience*, 15(5), 669–674.

[7] Job Accommodation Network (JAN). (2021). Accommodation and Compliance Series: Employees with Chronic Pain. U.S. Department of Labor, Office of Disability Employment Policy.

[8] Brown, B. (2012). *Daring Greatly: How the Courage to Be Vulnerable Transforms the Way We Live, Love, Parent, and Lead*. Gotham Books.

[9] Coan, J. A., & Sbarra, D. A. (2015). Social baseline theory: The social regulation of risk and effort. *Current Opinion in Psychology*, 1, 87–91.

Chapter Thirteen

Building Your Own Map Forward

When you picked up this book, you were probably carrying a lot. Confusion. Frustration. Maybe even anger or grief. You'd been repeatedly dismissed. Possibly misunderstood, or even told your pain wasn't real. You'd tried treatments that didn't work, visited providers who didn't listen, and gotten explanations that didn't make sense. The map you were given was incomplete. It doesn't matter if it was from medicine, society, or even your own personal history. And you were tired of being lost.

If you've made it this far, something has hopefully shifted. Maybe not in your pain, not yet, anyway. But in your understanding. You've learned that pain isn't just damage in the body but a signal interpreted by the nervous system. You've learned that maladaptive neuroplasticity isn't some abstract concept. It's the mechanism that explains why your pain moves, why it flares unpredictably, why no test captures it, and why you've felt gaslit for so long.

You've walked through the science. You've seen the interventions. You understand how movement, sleep, nervous system regulation, and trust-building work together to retrain a system that learned pain too well. And now you're standing at the edge of application. And you're probably wondering, what do I actually do with all of this?

That's what this final chapter is about. Not just what to do, but how to think about it. How to build your own map forward when the terrain is different for everyone. And how can you carry this framework into a life that won't always reinforce it. And finally, how to hold hope and realism in the same hand without letting either one slip.

This is not the end. It's the beginning.

The Framework You Now Carry

Let's start by naming what you now understand that you didn't know when you opened this book.

You understand that chronic pain isn't a life sentence handed down by faulty genes or bad luck. It's a learned state, a pattern your nervous system adopted in response to injury, illness, trauma, or prolonged stress. The system did its job. It protected you. But somewhere along the way, it learned too well. The alarm stayed on. The maps got redrawn. The signals got amplified. And pain became the default.[1]

You understand that these patterns aren't random. Fibromyalgia, EDS, CRPS, chronic infections, trauma-linked pain, they follow the same underlying logic rooted in central sensitization. Cortical remapping. Autonomic dysregulation. And trauma-encoded hypervigilance. The details differ, but the mechanism is the same. Your nervous system adapted, and now it needs to adapt again.[2]

You understand that this isn't about positive thinking or willpower. It's about inputs. The right movements, scaled correctly. Sleep that actually restores, and nervous system practices that shift you out of fight-or-flight. Tracking data that contradicts catastrophic predictions. As well as boundaries that protect your progress. These aren't optional add-ons, they're the language your nervous system understands.

And you understand that integration matters more than perfection. Movement reinforces trust. Sleep stabilizes the autonomic system, which makes movement safer. Nervous system regulation reduces hypervigilance, which improves sleep. Trust makes it easier to try new things, which generates more evidence, which deepens trust. The loop can work *for* you as powerfully as it once worked *against* you.[3]

This isn't just knowledge. It's a lens. And once you see through it, you can't unsee it.

Let me show you what this looks like in practice.

By the time you start this, you might be exhausted. Not just physically, but emotionally. You might have even stopped believing anything would work.

So you start small. Two chair squats, twice a week. That's it. No aggressive stretching, no high-intensity intervals, no push-through-the-pain mentality. Just two squats. You'll think you are wasting your time.

But within a few weeks, you'll notice something. The squats don't cause the flares you expected. Your legs feel steadier. You start adding a third squat, then a fourth. After a few more weeks, you're doing ten squats three times a week without consequence.

At the same time, you work on sleep. You adopt a consistent bedtime in a cooler room. You stop looking at screens an hour before bed, and begin journaling three wins from the day. Small inputs, repeated consistently. Your sleep improves from four fragmented hours to six more solid ones. And when you sleep better, the pain is quieter the next day. Movement feels easier. The catastrophic thoughts are less frequent.

You add breathwork, just five minutes of diaphragmatic breathing when you feel your nervous system ramping up. Then you start tracking your flares in a journal. What triggered them, how intense, how long, and what helped. Over time, you notice patterns. Social stress is a bigger trigger than physical activity. Late-night scrolling spikes your pain the next morning. When you address those inputs, your flares shorten.

Six months in, you're not pain-free. But your flares go from weekly to monthly. They last three days instead of two weeks. You can walk your dog again. You can make plans without the crushing anxiety that you might have to cancel. And most importantly, you trust your body again. Not because it's perfect, but because you understand it.

That's integration. It's not just one magic intervention. It's multiple small inputs working together over time. Each piece reinforces the others, and the nervous system slowly learns a new pattern.

What "Better" Actually Means

Let's be honest about something. This work doesn't always lead to "cured." And that's okay. Because "better" doesn't have to mean pain-free to be worth it.

For some people, better means a significant reduction in their pain. For example, pain that was an 8 out of 10 becomes a 3. For others, it means predictability, or knowing what triggers flares and being able to manage them. For some, it's reclaiming activities they thought were gone forever. And for others, it's just getting through the day without catastrophizing every sensation.

All of these are valid. All of these are successes.

The dominant narrative around chronic pain recovery is either "you're cured" or "you're failing." That's bullshit. Recovery is a spectrum, and where you land depends on many factors. Factors such as how long you've been in pain, what other conditions you're managing, what resources you have access to, how much support you get, and, yes, some degree of variability in how individual nervous systems respond.

Here's what research on long-term pain outcomes actually shows. Most people who engage in multimodal pain management, such as nervous system retraining and graded movement exposure, see meaningful improvement. Not elimination, but reduction. Not perfection, but function. Not a return to "before," but a reclamation of life.[4]

What Progress Looks Like Over Time

Three months in:

You're starting to see patterns. Flares are still happening, but they're slightly shorter or less intense. You've had a few wins. It may be a movement that didn't cause disaster, or a night of decent sleep. Or it could even be a day where pain wasn't the loudest thing in your awareness. You're not sure if it's working yet, but you're willing to keep trying.

Six months in:

The changes are undeniable. Flares are less frequent. Recovery is faster. You've reclaimed small activities. You can now walk to the mailbox or cook a simple meal. You can sit through a movie without needing to shift every five minutes. And you're tracking data that shows progress, even when it doesn't feel like progress. Trust is building.

One year in:

Pain is no longer the main event. It's background noise. Some days it's louder, other days quieter. But it doesn't define your day anymore. You've had setbacks. But you know how to navigate them. You make plans without calculating whether your body can handle them. You trust the process because you've seen it work.

Two years and beyond:

You're living. Not just managing, but actually living. Pain might still be there, but it's not in the driver's seat. You've rebuilt trust in your body. You've learned what your system needs. And you've reclaimed enough function that life feels worth engaging with again.

This isn't a guarantee. But it's a possibility. And possibility is what this book is offering.

Building Your Personal Map

Integration gives you the framework. Now you need to build your own map: the specific practices, routines, and tools that make sense for your body, your condition, and your life.

Here's the thing. Your map will look different from someone else's. The person with fibromyalgia will prioritize differently from the person with EDS. The person with PTSD-linked pain will need different inputs than the person with Long COVID. And that's okay. The principles are universal, and the application is personal.

Start With One Entry Point

Don't try to overhaul everything at once. Pick one entry point. Pick the intervention that feels most accessible or most urgent, and start there.

If sleep is your biggest struggle:

Start with sleep hygiene. Keep a consistent bedtime and a cooler room. Stay away from screens before bed, and practice your wind-down ritual. Give it two weeks of consistent practice before adding anything else. Sleep stabilizes downstream processes, including pain thresholds, emotional regulation, and cognitive function. If you improve sleep, movement, and nervous system work gets easier.[5]

If movement feels impossible:

Start with the smallest tolerable dose. Do one movement, repeated consistently. Chair squats. Arm raises. Walking to the mailbox. The goal isn't intensity, it's consistency. The nervous system learns through repetition, not heroics.[6]

If your nervous system is stuck in high alert:

Start with regulation practices. Diaphragmatic breathing. Grounding exercises. Short body scans. These don't fix pain directly, but they shift you out of fight-or-flight. And this can make everything else easier.[7]

If trust is shattered:

Start with tracking. Write down one thing that went better than expected each day. Just one. This creates evidence that contradicts catastrophic predictions. And evidence is what trust needs to grow.[8]

Pick one. Master it. Let it stabilize. Then add the next piece.

Build Your Personal Protocol

Once you have one entry point stabilized, you can start layering in other practices. Here's a framework for building your protocol:

Foundation layer (daily non-negotiables):

• Sleep: consistent bedtime, sleep-supportive environment

• Baseline movement: whatever you can do consistently without flaring

• Nervous system check-in: one practice that shifts you toward parasympathetic (breath, grounding, etc.)

Progressive layer (things you scale up over time):

- Movement intensity: add reps, add frequency, add range of motion

- Activity reclamation: reintroduce one meaningful activity at a time

- Social engagement: dose your energy strategically

Adaptive layer (things you adjust based on context):

- Pacing strategies: how you manage high-demand days

- Flare protocols: what you do when symptoms spike

- Boundary setting: how you protect your progress in challenging situations

Your protocol isn't fixed. It adapts with you. What works at three months might not be what you need at six months. What you prioritize during a flare might look different than what you do during a stable period. The map evolves.

Track What Matters

You can't know what's working if you're not tracking it. But don't track everything, that's overwhelming. Track the things that give you useful information.

Track your inputs:

What did you do? Movement, sleep quality, nervous system practices, and social energy expenditure. Keep it simple. A sentence or two per day is enough.

Track your outputs:

How did your body respond? What were your pain levels (0-10 scale)? Then track your energy levels, mood, and function. Again, keep it simple. You're looking for patterns, not perfection.

Track your wins:

What went better than expected? This is the most important metric because it builds trust. "Walked to the mailbox without bracing." "Slept six hours." "Caught a catastrophic thought and reframed it." These matter.

Over time, the data tells you what's working. And when you hit a rough patch, you can look back and see evidence of progress even when it doesn't feel like progress in the moment.

Adjust Based on Feedback

Your body is constantly giving you feedback. The question is whether you're listening to it accurately.

If something consistently causes flares, scale it back. You're asking too much too soon. Find a smaller version of the same input and build from there. If something used to help but stopped working, you might have plateaued. Add variation. Try different movement patterns, times of day, or intensities. The nervous system needs novelty to keep adapting. If you're improving in one area but stuck in another, look for connections. Sleep improved, but movement still causes flares? Your nervous system might still be interpreting movement as a threat. Add more grounding before and after movement sessions. Lastly, if progress stalls completely, step back and reassess. Are you missing a piece? Sleep, stress, trauma, social support, and medical factors? Sometimes progress requires addressing something you haven't yet prioritized.

Your map isn't static. It's a living document that changes with you.

The Compass You Carry Forward

Maps show you where you are. Compasses show you where you're going. And the compass you carry forward has four cardinal directions: Safety, Adaptation, Agency, and Hope.

North: Safety

Every decision you make should point toward safety. Not just physical safety, but nervous system safety. Does this input help my system feel less threatened? Does this relationship support my healing or undermine it? Does this environment allow me to regulate my hypervigilance or push me into it? When you're lost or don't know what to do next, orient toward safety. Ask yourself, what would make my nervous system feel safer right now? Sometimes that's movement. Sometimes it's rest. Sometimes it's a boundary. Sometimes it's a connection. But safety is always the direction that moves you forward.[9]

East: Adaptation

Your nervous system adapted into pain. It can adapt out. Every practice you engage with is teaching your system something new. The question is, what are you teaching it? When you move despite fear, you teach it that movement is safe. When you sleep consistently, you teach it that rest is possible. When you track wins, you teach it that progress is real. Adaptation happens through repetition, not perfection. Point your compass toward small, consistent inputs that teach the system new patterns.[10]

South: Agency

Agency is the sense that your actions matter, that you have influence over outcomes, and that you're steering your own ship. Chronic pain strips that away. It makes the body feel like an enemy, unpredictable and untrustworthy. And when the world dismisses your experience, it reinforces that loss of control. Reclaiming it is part of healing. When you're overwhelmed, point your compass toward agency. What's one small thing I can control right now? Not everything. Just one thing. It could be choosing to rest instead of pushing through. Perhaps it could be setting a boundary. Maybe it's trying one graded movement. Each small act of agency reinforces the pathway that you are not helpless. You have influence. Your choices matter.[11]

West: Hope

Hope isn't about believing everything will be perfect. It's about accepting that change is possible. And hope grounded not in wishful thinking but in actual neurological possibility is powerful. When doubt creeps in, point your compass toward hope. Not blind optimism, but evidence-based possibility. Your nervous system is plastic. What was learned can be unlearned. Progress is happening even when you can't see it. Others have walked this path. You're not alone. This is hard, but it's not impossible.

The compass doesn't make the terrain easy. But it keeps you oriented. And orientation is what allows you to keep moving forward even when the path isn't clear.

Navigating the Path Ahead

You have the framework. You have the tools. Now let's talk about the reality of walking this path in a world that won't always support you.

Finding Care That Aligns

Not every provider understands neuroplastic pain. In fact, most don't. This is frustrating, but it doesn't mean you can't make progress.

If you can find a provider who gets it, like a pain specialist, a physical therapist, or a therapist who understands trauma and chronic pain, hold onto them.

Good providers are out there. And when you find one, they're worth their weight in gold.

But if you can't find that provider, whether it's because of geography, finances, insurance limitations, or just bad luck, you can still move forward. The framework in this book gives you enough to work with. You might not have perfect guidance, but you have direction. And direction is enough to start.

When working with providers who don't fully understand this lens, you can still get value from them. A physical therapist who doesn't know about central sensitization can still help you scale movement appropriately if you communicate your needs clearly. A doctor who doesn't understand maladaptive neuroplasticity can still order tests to rule out other factors. You don't need them to share your framework; you just need them to respect your experience and collaborate with you.

If a provider dismisses you, invalidates you, or refuses to work with you as a partner, you have permission to walk away. Not every relationship is worth saving, and your healing is more important than their ego.

When You Can't Afford "Perfect" Care

Let's be real. A lot of the interventions that help with chronic pain aren't covered by insurance. Manual therapy, specialized physical therapy, and trauma-informed therapy often require out-of-pocket payment that not everyone can manage.

If you can't afford ideal care, here's what you can still do:

Movement: Free. You don't need a gym membership or fancy equipment. Chair squats, wall sits, and gentle stretching. You can do all of this at home.

Sleep hygiene: Free. Consistent bedtimes, cooler rooms, and wind-down rituals. None of this costs money.

Nervous system regulation: Free. Breathing exercises, grounding practices, and body scans. All of these are accessible without spending a dime.

Tracking: Free. A notebook and a pen are all you need to track inputs, outputs, and wins.

Community: Mostly free. Online support groups, forums, and advocacy spaces. These offer connection and shared knowledge without cost.

The interventions that matter most are the ones you can do consistently. And most of those don't require money. They require time, attention, and patience. If you have those, you have enough to start.

Maintaining Progress Without Perfect Support

You don't need a team of specialists to maintain progress. You need a few things:

Consistency. Small inputs, repeated over time, accumulate into change.

Feedback loops. Track what's working, adjust what isn't, keep moving forward.

Boundaries. Protect your progress from people and environments that undermine it.

Community. Connect with others who understand, even if it's just online.

Self-compassion. This is hard work. You're allowed to struggle. You're allowed to have setbacks. And you're allowed to keep going anyway.[12]

Perfect support would be nice. But you don't need perfect. You just need enough.

Working Within Broken Systems

The medical system is not set up to support complex chronic pain. Insurance doesn't cover what helps most. Providers are overworked and undertrained. Wait times are long. Access is unequal. This isn't fair, and it's not your fault.

You can't fix the system. But you can navigate it strategically.

Document everything. Keep records of symptoms, treatments tried, and provider interactions. This protects you if you need to advocate for accommodations or appeal insurance decisions.

Learn the language. Medical systems respond to specific terminology. "Central sensitization," "maladaptive neuroplasticity," and "nociplastic pain" are terms that can help you communicate with providers who understand them.

Ask for what you need. Be specific. "I need a referral to a pain specialist who understands central sensitization" is more effective than "I need help with my pain."

Build a backup plan. If insurance won't cover something, what's your alternative? Online resources?

Community support? Self-directed practice? Always have a Plan B.

The system is broken. But you're not. And you can make progress despite the system, not because of it.

What You're Reclaiming

This book has focused a lot on pain management. But here's what you're actually doing: you're reclaiming your life and your agency. Reclaiming agency doesn't mean controlling the pain. It means controlling your response to it. It means making choices that honor your nervous system's needs rather than other people's expectations. It means recognizing that you are the expert on your own body, even when the world thinks otherwise.

Small acts of agency build over time:

Choosing to rest when you're tired, even when someone else thinks you should push through. Setting a boundary, even when it feels uncomfortable. Tracking your wins, even when they feel too small to matter. Deciding what treatments to try, based on your own research and intuition, not just provider recommendations. And saying no to events, people, or obligations that don't serve your healing. Each act is a declaration: I am in charge of my own healing. That doesn't mean you're alone in this. It means you're the one steering the ship.

Identity Beyond Pain

When pain has been your reality for years, your identity fuses with it. You become "the sick one," "the person who can't," or "the one who's always in pain." And when that's your primary identity, improvement feels threatening. If you're not in pain, who are you?

Part of healing is rebuilding identity separate from pain. Not instead of acknowledging pain, but alongside it. You're more than your diagnosis. You're more than your symptoms. And reclaiming that truth is part of the work.

Who were you before pain took over? What did you care about? What brought you joy? What made you feel alive? Some of those things might not be accessible in the same way anymore. But some version of them probably is.

Maybe you loved hiking, and now you can't. But you can sit by a trail and watch the light through the trees. Maybe you loved cooking elaborate meals, and now you can't stand for that long. But perhaps you can make one simple dish that brings you pleasure. Maybe you loved being the person everyone leaned on, and now you can't carry that weight. But you can offer something smaller, such as a kind word, a listening ear, a moment of presence.

Identity isn't about going back to who you were. It's about discovering who you're becoming. And that person, the one who's walked through this fire and is still standing, is someone worth knowing.[13]

Purpose and Meaning Beyond Survival

For a long time, survival was the goal. Getting through the day, managing the pain, and making it to the next appointment. And survival is important. But it's not the same as living.

As you reclaim function, you reclaim the capacity to think beyond survival. What do you actually want? What matters to you? What would make your life feel meaningful, not just manageable?

These are hard questions, especially when you've been in survival mode for years. But they're worth sitting with. Because healing isn't just about reducing pain, it's about building a life that feels worth living.

That could be reconnecting with old passions. Maybe it's discovering new ones. It could be contributing to your community in small ways. Perhaps it's just being present for the people you love without pain dominating every interaction. Whatever it is, it's yours to define.

Holding Grief and Hope Together

Let's be honest here, Chronic pain takes things from you. Time. Relationships. Opportunities. The life you thought you'd have. And it's okay to grieve that. You don't have to pretend it's fine. You don't have to silver-lining it away.

But grief and hope aren't mutually exclusive. You can mourn what was lost and still believe that something meaningful is possible in the future. You can acknowledge the unfairness of your situation and still choose to engage with the tools that help. You can be angry at what chronic pain took from you and still show up for the life you're building now.

Both can be true. And holding them both is part of what it means to live with chronic pain in a realistic, sustainable way.[14]

You Are Not Alone

One of the most isolating parts of chronic pain is feeling like no one else understands. Like you're navigating this alone. Like everyone else has it figured out, and you're the only one still struggling.

That's not true.

There are millions of people living with chronic pain. Thousands who've walked the path you're walking now. Hundreds who are reading this book alongside you, asking the same questions, feeling the same fears, hoping for the same possibility.

You're not alone. And finding your people, the ones who get it without needing explanation, can be one of the most healing parts of this journey.

Finding (and Being) Your People

You don't have to do this alone. And while the world at large may not understand, some people do.

Some of them are in chronic pain communities, such as online forums, support groups, and advocacy spaces, where the language of scaling, pacing, and nervous system recalibration isn't foreign. It's home.

Others are individuals you'll find along the way. A provider who listens. A friend who doesn't need you to justify your limits. A family member who learns, slowly, how to support you without fixing you.

These people matter. Not because they validate your experience. You don't need external validation to know your pain is real. But because they reduce the cost of being seen. You don't have to translate. You don't have to defend. You can just be, and that's enough.

Online communities:

Reddit, Facebook groups, and patient advocacy organizations. Look for communities that balance validation with forward movement. If every post is despair with no room for progress, keep looking. But communities that acknowledge the reality of chronic pain while also supporting each other's healing? Those are gold.

Local support groups:

Check with hospitals, pain clinics, and community health centers. In-person connection combats isolation in ways virtual connection can't fully replicate.

Therapists who specialize in chronic pain:

Not all therapists understand chronic pain, but the ones who do are invaluable. They can help you process the grief, navigate the identity shifts, and manage the emotional weight without needing you to explain yourself.

Practitioners who listen:

Good providers exist. When you find one who believes you, who collaborates with you, who respects your experience, hold onto them.

How to Be Good Support for Others

If you're in a position to support someone else with chronic pain, here's what helps:

Believe them. Even if you don't understand. Even if their pain seems disproportionate. Even if their limits frustrate you.

Don't offer unsolicited advice. They've probably already tried what you're suggesting.

Respect their limits without guilt-tripping. If they cancel plans, just say, "No problem, let me know when you're up for it."

Celebrate small wins. They matter, even when they seem invisible to you.

Don't compare. "I get tired too" isn't supportive. It's dismissive.

Being good support doesn't require you to fully understand chronic pain. It just requires you to believe the person in front of you and respect their reality.

The Beginning

This book opened with confusion, pain that felt senseless, dismissed, and isolating. It walked you through the science of how pain works, how the nervous system learns maladaptive patterns, and how seemingly mysterious conditions share the same underlying mechanisms. It gave you tools like movement, sleep, regulation, trust-building, boundaries, and integration.

But the real work starts now.

You're not broken. You never were. You're living with a nervous system that adapted too well and needs to adapt again. That adaptation won't happen overnight. It won't be linear. There will be setbacks. There will be days when it feels impossible. But every small input you provide, every movement, every boundary, every moment of regulation, is teaching your system something new.

Progress isn't about perfection. It's about direction. And you have direction now. You have a framework that explains what felt inexplicable. You have tools that work with your nervous system, not against it. You have a compass that keeps you oriented even when the path isn't clear.

The map forward is yours to draw. You know the terrain better than anyone. You know what your body needs, what your life can hold, and what progress looks like for you. No one else can draw this map. But you're not drawing it alone.

Thousands of people have walked this path before you. Thousands are walking it alongside you right now. And thousands more will walk it after you, guided in part by the path you're carving.

This is not the end. It's the beginning. The knowledge you gained from this book is the foundation. The practices you build from here are the structure. And the life you reclaim is the proof that adaptation is possible.

You are not broken. You are adaptable. And adaptability means there's always a way forward.

One breath at a time. One movement at a time. One day at a time.

You've got this.

Final Reflection

Before you close this book, take a moment to sit with these questions:

What have I learned that changes how I see my pain?

Which practice feels most sustainable for me to carry forward tomorrow?

What's one small action I can take this week to start building my map?

How will I remind myself that progress is built from small wins, not giant leaps?

What will I tell my future self a year from now?

Your answers are your starting point. They're the first landmarks on your map. Let them guide you.

The compass is in your hands now. The terrain is yours to navigate. The story you write from here, that's yours too.

And it starts today.

Endnotes

[1] Moseley, G. L., & Butler, D. S. (2015). Fifteen years of explaining pain: The past, present, and future. *Journal of Pain*, 16(9), 807–813.

[2] Nijs, J., Leysen, L., Vanlauwe, J., Logghe, T., Ickmans, K., Polli, A., Malfliet, A., Coppieters, I., & Huysmans, E. (2019). Treatment of central sensitization in patients with chronic pain: Time for change? *Expert Opinion on Pharmacotherapy*, 20(16), 1961–1970.

[3] Moseley, G. L., & Flor, H. (2012). Targeting cortical representations in the treatment of chronic pain: A review. *Neurorehabilitation and Neural Repair*, 26(6), 646–652.

[4] Kamper, S. J., Apeldoorn, A. T., Chiarotto, A., et al. (2015). Multidisciplinary biopsychosocial rehabilitation for chronic low back pain. *Cochrane Database of Systematic Reviews*, (9), CD000963.

[5] Finan, P. H., Goodin, B. R., & Smith, M. T. (2013). The association of sleep and pain: An update and a path forward. *The Journal of Pain*, 14(12), 1539–1552.

[6] Booth, J., Moseley, G. L., Schiltenwolf, M., Cashin, A., Davies, M., & Hübscher, M. (2017). Exercise for chronic musculoskeletal pain: A biopsychosocial approach. *Musculoskeletal Care*, 15(4), 413–421.

[7] Porges, S. W. (2011). *The Polyvagal Theory: Neurophysiological Foundations of Emotions, Attachment, Communication, and Self-regulation*. W. W. Norton & Company.

[8] Jackson, T., Wang, Y., Wang, Y., & Fan, H. (2014). Self-efficacy and chronic pain outcomes: A meta-analytic review. *The Journal of Pain*, 15(8), 800–814.

[9] Brown, C. A., & Jones, A. K. P. (2010). Meditation experience predicts less negative appraisal of pain: Electrophysiological support for the mindfulness–stress buffering account. Pain, 150(3), 428–439.

[10] Moseley, G. L. (2004). Evidence for a direct relationship between cognitive and physical change during an education intervention in chronic pain. Pain, 109(1–2), 37–45.

[11] Bandura, A. (1997). *Self-efficacy: The exercise of control*. W.H. Freeman and Company.

[12] Neff, K. D. (2003). Self-compassion: An alternative conceptualization of a healthy attitude toward oneself. *Self and Identity*, 2(2), 85–101.

[13] Charmaz, K. (1983). Loss of self: A fundamental form of suffering in the chronically ill. *Sociology of Health & Illness*, 5(2), 168–195.

[14] McCracken, L. M., & Vowles, K. E. (2014). Acceptance and Commitment Therapy and mindfulness for chronic pain: Model, process, and progress. *American Psychologist*, 69(2), 178–187.

Glossary of Terms

A

Acute Pain

Pain that arises suddenly in response to tissue damage or injury and typically resolves as healing occurs. Acute pain serves a protective function, alerting you to harm and encouraging rest or treatment. Unlike chronic pain, it follows predictable patterns and diminishes with recovery.

Agency

The sense that your actions matter and that you have influence over outcomes. Chronic pain strips agency by making the body feel unpredictable and untrustworthy. Rebuilding agency means reclaiming small, concrete choices—resting when you need to, setting boundaries, choosing which inputs you practice—that reinforce "I am not helpless. I have influence over my healing."

Allodynia

A condition in which normally non-painful stimuli produce pain. For example, light touch, clothing against the skin, or a gentle breeze may feel painful.

Allodynia results from central sensitization, where the nervous system has become hypersensitive and misinterprets ordinary sensations as threats.

Amygdala

An almond-shaped structure deep in the brain's limbic system that functions as the brain's primary threat detector. The amygdala processes fear, emotional responses, and memory consolidation related to threatening experiences. In chronic pain, the amygdala can become hypervigilant, interpreting normal sensations as dangerous and amplifying pain signals.

Anterior Cingulate Cortex (ACC)

A brain region involved in processing the emotional and motivational aspects of pain. The ACC determines how much pain *matters*—transforming sensation into suffering. Research shows heightened ACC activity in people with chronic pain, especially when they feel hopeless or catastrophize about their symptoms.

Autonomic Nervous System

The branch of the nervous system that regulates automatic bodily functions like heart rate, blood pressure, digestion, breathing, and temperature. It consists of two divisions: the sympathetic nervous system (fight-or-flight) and the parasympathetic nervous system (rest-and-digest). In chronic pain, the autonomic system often becomes dysregulated, stuck in sympathetic overdrive.

B

Baseline (Activity Baseline)
The level of activity you can do consistently, day after day, without triggering a flare or crash. Your baseline is usually lower than you think and lower than what you can do on a "good day." Pacing and graded activity rely on finding and respecting this baseline, then building from it slowly.

Baseline Movement
The minimum, sustainable amount of movement you aim to do daily (or most days), even when symptoms are present. This might be as simple as a short walk, a few chair squats, or gentle range-of-motion work. The goal is consistency, not intensity, so the nervous system learns that movement is safe and predictable.

Blood Sugar Stability
A state where blood glucose doesn't swing wildly between spikes and crashes throughout the day. Unstable blood sugar triggers stress hormones like cortisol and adrenaline, which can keep the nervous

system in a low-grade fight-or-flight state and lower pain thresholds. Eating in ways that avoid big spikes and crashes removes one avoidable stressor from an already overloaded system.

Body Map (See also: Cortical Body Map)
The brain's internal representation of the physical body. These maps exist in the somatosensory cortex and organize sensory information by body region. When these maps become distorted through injury, trauma, or chronic pain, the brain may misinterpret signals, creating pain in areas where no tissue damage exists.

Brain Fog
A colloquial term for cognitive difficulties including impaired concentration, memory problems, mental fatigue, and slowed thinking. Common in chronic pain conditions like fibromyalgia, EDS, and ME/CFS, brain fog results from nervous system overload and the constant cognitive demand of managing pain and bodily dysfunction.

Breathing Techniques
Deliberate ways of changing your breathing pattern to influence nervous system state. Examples in this book include diaphragmatic breathing and 4-7-8 breathing. These techniques work by stimulating the

parasympathetic nervous system, slowing heart rate, lowering arousal, and sending a "we're safe" signal upstream to the brain.

C

Catastrophizing
A cognitive pattern where someone focuses on the worst possible outcomes of their pain, magnifies its threat, and feels helpless to manage it. Catastrophizing amplifies pain perception through increased limbic system activation and can predict worse pain outcomes. It's not weakness or exaggeration—it's a learned cognitive response that can be retrained.

Central Nervous System (CNS)
The brain and spinal cord. The CNS processes all sensory information, coordinates responses, and generates conscious experience. In chronic pain, the CNS can become sensitized, amplifying pain signals independently of peripheral tissue damage.

Central Sensitization
A state in which the central nervous system becomes hypersensitive to stimulation, amplifying pain signals and lowering pain thresholds. With central

sensitization, the nervous system is "stuck" in high alert, interpreting even normal or mild sensations as painful. This process involves neural plasticity—the nervous system learns to produce pain more efficiently and struggles to turn it off.

Chronic Fatigue Syndrome (See: Myalgic Encephalomyelitis/Chronic Fatigue Syndrome)

Chronic Pain
Pain that persists beyond the normal healing time (typically longer than three to six months) or recurs over months or years. Unlike acute pain, chronic pain often serves no protective function and may persist even after tissue healing is complete. Chronic pain involves changes in the nervous system itself, including central sensitization and cortical reorganization.

Circadian Rhythm
The body's internal 24-hour clock that regulates sleep–wake cycles, hormone release, temperature, and many other functions. Light exposure, meal timing, and routine strongly influence circadian rhythms. When they're disrupted, sleep quality drops, pain sensitivity increases, and the nervous system has a harder time accessing restorative states.

Cognitive-Behavioral Therapy (CBT)

A therapeutic approach that addresses the relationship between thoughts, emotions, and behaviors. In pain management, CBT helps patients recognize and reframe catastrophic thinking, reduce fear-avoidance, and develop coping strategies. CBT doesn't claim pain is imaginary—it works by reducing the emotional amplification that worsens pain perception.

Cognitive-Behavioral Therapy for Insomnia (CBT-I)

A specific form of CBT designed to treat insomnia. CBT-I targets patterns of thought and behavior that keep people stuck in poor sleep: spending too long in bed awake, associating bed with worry, erratic sleep schedules, and anxiety about sleep itself. It has strong evidence for improving sleep quality long term without relying solely on medication.

Collagen

A structural protein that provides strength and elasticity to connective tissues throughout the body, including skin, ligaments, tendons, and blood vessels. In Ehlers-Danlos Syndrome, genetic mutations affect collagen production or structure, leading to tissue fragility, joint hypermobility, and other complications.

Complex Regional Pain Syndrome (CRPS)

A chronic pain condition typically triggered by an

injury, surgery, or trauma to a limb. CRPS is characterized by severe, burning pain disproportionate to the initial injury, along with changes in skin color, temperature, and swelling. The condition involves both peripheral and central nervous system changes, including altered cortical body maps and inflammatory processes. Previously known as Reflex Sympathetic Dystrophy (RSD).

Comorbidity

The presence of two or more medical conditions occurring together in the same person. Many chronic pain conditions cluster together (fibromyalgia with EDS, POTS with MCAS, etc.), suggesting shared underlying mechanisms rather than random coincidence.

Connective Tissue

Biological tissue that supports, connects, or separates different types of tissues and organs in the body. It includes bone, cartilage, ligaments, tendons, and fascia. In Ehlers-Danlos Syndrome, defects in connective tissue lead to joint instability, tissue fragility, and chronic pain.

Cortical Body Map (See also: Somatosensory Cortex)

The brain's organized representation of the body's surface and internal structures, located primarily in the somatosensory cortex. These maps are not fixed—they reorganize based on experience, injury, and use. In chronic pain, these maps can become distorted, enlarged, or blurred, causing the brain to misinterpret signals and generate pain in areas without tissue damage.

Cortical Reorganization

The process by which the brain's cortical maps change in response to experience, injury, or altered sensory input. In chronic pain, cortical reorganization often involves enlargement or distortion of painful body regions' representations, leading to amplified and spreading pain. This reorganization can be reversed through targeted interventions.

Cortisol

A primary stress hormone released by the adrenal glands. Short-term cortisol spikes help you respond to danger. Chronically elevated cortisol, however, disrupts sleep, keeps the body in high alert, impairs immune function, and lowers pain thresholds. In many chronic pain states, cortisol patterns are flattened or chronically elevated, feeding the pain loop.

Cytokines

Small signaling proteins released by immune cells (and glial cells in the nervous system) that coordinate inflammatory responses. In chronic pain and conditions like fibromyalgia or ME/CFS, low-grade, ongoing cytokine activity contributes to neuroinflammation, fatigue, and increased pain sensitivity.

D

Deep Sleep (Slow-Wave Sleep)
The most restorative stage of non-REM sleep (also called N3 or slow-wave sleep). During this stage, growth hormone is released, tissue repair occurs, the glymphatic system clears metabolic waste from the brain, and pain thresholds reset. Chronic disruption of deep sleep is a major driver of increased pain sensitivity and fatigue.

Default Mode Network (DMN)
A network of brain regions that becomes active during rest, mind-wandering, and self-referential thinking. In chronic pain and trauma, the DMN can become hyperactive, leading to rumination, catastrophizing, and excessive self-monitoring. Mindfulness practices help quiet the DMN.

Descending Inhibition (See also: Descending Modulation)

The brain's ability to send signals down the spinal cord that reduce or block incoming pain signals. This is part of the body's natural pain control system. In chronic pain, descending inhibition often becomes impaired, allowing more pain signals to reach the brain. Certain interventions (like exercise, mindfulness, and some medications) can strengthen descending inhibition.

Descending Modulation

The brain's active regulation of pain signals traveling from the body. The brain can either amplify (descending facilitation) or dampen (descending inhibition) pain signals before they fully register. Stress, fear, and catastrophizing activate descending facilitation, while relaxation, safety, and positive expectation activate descending inhibition.

Diaphragmatic Breathing

A breathing pattern that emphasizes slow, deep breaths driven by the diaphragm rather than shallow chest breathing. The belly rises on inhalation and falls on exhalation. Diaphragmatic breathing stimulates the vagus nerve and parasympathetic nervous system, lowering arousal, reducing muscle tension, and helping interrupt the pain–stress loop.

Dysautonomia
Dysfunction of the autonomic nervous system, affecting regulation of heart rate, blood pressure, digestion, temperature, and other automatic functions. Common in POTS, EDS, fibromyalgia, and ME/CFS. Symptoms include dizziness, fainting, rapid heartbeat, digestive issues, and temperature regulation problems.

E

Ehlers-Danlos Syndrome (EDS)
A group of genetic connective tissue disorders characterized by joint hypermobility, skin hyperextensibility, and tissue fragility. The hypermobile type (hEDS) is most common and often involves chronic pain, fatigue, proprioceptive deficits, and comorbid conditions like POTS, MCAS, and dysautonomia. Pain in EDS is driven not just by structural instability but also by altered cortical body maps and central sensitization.

Endogenous Opioids
The body's natural pain-relieving chemicals, including endorphins, enkephalins, and dynorphins. These bind to opioid receptors in the brain and spinal cord,

reducing pain perception. The placebo effect often works by triggering the release of endogenous opioids.

Exposure Therapy

A therapeutic approach where someone gradually confronts feared situations or activities in a controlled, safe manner. In pain management, graded exposure involves slowly increasing movement or activity despite pain-related fear, teaching the nervous system that the activity is safe and recalibrating threat responses.

F

Fear-Avoidance

A cycle where fear of pain leads to avoidance of movement or activity, which increases deconditioning, disability, and paradoxically worsens pain over time. The fear-avoidance model explains how psychological factors contribute to chronic pain disability. Breaking this cycle through graded exposure is a key intervention strategy.

Fibromyalgia

A chronic condition characterized by widespread pain, fatigue, sleep disturbances, cognitive difficulties ("fibro fog"), and heightened sensitivity to sensory stimuli. Fibromyalgia represents central sensitization in its most pronounced form—the nervous system stuck in overdrive, amplifying signals until everything feels threatening. Research shows altered pain processing, impaired descending inhibition, and dysregulated stress responses.

Fight-or-Flight Response

The body's acute stress response, activated by the sympathetic nervous system when threat is detected. This response increases heart rate, blood pressure, muscle tension, and stress hormone release while suppressing non-essential functions like digestion. In chronic pain, this system often becomes chronically activated, perpetuating pain and preventing recovery.

Flare / Flare-Up

A temporary spike or worsening of symptoms—pain, fatigue, brain fog, dysautonomia—often triggered by overexertion, stress, poor sleep, illness, or sensory overload. Flares are part of the pattern of chronic pain conditions. They don't mean permanent damage, but they do signal that the system has been pushed beyond its current capacity.

G

Gate Control Theory

A landmark theory of pain proposed by Melzack and Wall in 1965, suggesting that pain signals must pass through a "gate" in the spinal cord before reaching the brain. This gate can be opened (allowing more pain signals through) or closed (blocking pain signals) by various factors including other sensory input, emotional state, and descending signals from the brain. This theory revolutionized pain science by showing that pain is actively modulated, not just passively transmitted.

Glycine

An amino acid sometimes used as a supplement to support sleep and, in some contexts, connective tissue health. Taken before bed (for example, 3 grams), it may modestly improve sleep onset and subjective sleep quality, which indirectly supports pain management by improving recovery.

Glymphatic System

The brain's waste-clearance system, most active during deep sleep. Cerebrospinal fluid flushes metabolic byproducts and inflammatory waste out of brain tissue. When deep sleep is chronically disrupted, glymphatic clearance suffers, contributing to fatigue, cognitive problems, and possibly increased pain sensitivity.

Glial Cells
Non-neuronal cells in the brain and spinal cord that support and regulate neurons. In chronic pain, glial cells can become activated and release inflammatory chemicals that sensitize pain pathways, contributing to central sensitization and neuroinflammation.

Graded Activity
A rehabilitation approach where activity levels are gradually and systematically increased over time, regardless of pain levels. The goal is to prevent boom-bust cycles, rebuild tolerance, and teach the nervous system that movement is safe. Pacing is key—finding a sustainable baseline and building slowly.

Graded Exposure (See: Exposure Therapy)

Graded Motor Imagery (GMI)
A therapeutic technique that uses mental imagery of movement to retrain the brain's motor and sensory maps without actual movement. GMI has been shown effective in conditions like CRPS, phantom limb pain, and chronic pain where movement itself has become threatening. The technique works through

neuroplasticity, allowing the brain to reorganize without triggering protective pain responses.

Grounding

Simple practices that anchor attention in the present moment and in the body: feeling your feet on the floor, noticing the contact of your back with a chair, naming things you can see/hear/feel. Grounding reduces limbic over-activation and helps the nervous system shift out of spiraling threat states.

H

Hippocampus

A brain structure in the limbic system crucial for memory formation, spatial navigation, and contextualizing experiences. The hippocampus helps distinguish past from present ("this hurt before" vs. "this always hurts"). Chronic stress, trauma, and pain can impair hippocampal function, making it harder to update threat associations and contributing to persistent fear responses.

Hyperalgesia

An exaggerated pain response to stimuli that are normally only mildly painful. For example, a small bump or light pressure produces intense, prolonged pain. Hyperalgesia results from central sensitization, where the nervous system amplifies pain signals beyond normal levels.

Hypermobility

Excessive range of motion in joints, often called being "double-jointed." While some degree of hypermobility is common and benign, in Ehlers-Danlos Syndrome it results from defective collagen and can lead to chronic pain, instability, dislocations, and proprioceptive deficits. Many people with hypermobility are dismissed as it looks impressive or flexible, but it creates constant demand on muscles to stabilize unstable joints.

Hypervigilance

A state of chronic, heightened alertness where the nervous system constantly scans for threat. Hypervigilance can apply to external threats (sounds, people, environments) or internal sensations (heart rate, pain, dizziness). In chronic pain, hypervigilance makes every sensation feel suspicious and keeps the system primed for flare-ups.

Hydration

Adequate fluid balance in the body. Dehydration lowers blood volume, reduces tissue oxygenation, increases muscle tightness, and can lower pain thresholds.

Staying reasonably hydrated is a simple way to remove an extra stressor from an already overloaded nervous system.

I

Inflammation
The body's immune response to injury or infection, involving swelling, heat, redness, and pain. While acute inflammation is protective and promotes healing, chronic low-grade inflammation can sensitize pain pathways. In conditions like CRPS and some cases of ME/CFS, inflammatory processes contribute to pain and symptom persistence.

Insula
A brain region tucked deep within the cortex that processes interoception—awareness of the body's internal state. The insula tracks heart rate, breathing, temperature, gut sensations, and pain. In chronic pain, the insula often becomes hyperactive, leading to excessive body monitoring and amplification of internal signals. This contributes to the feeling of being "too aware" of your body.

Interoception
The sense of the body's internal state, including hunger, thirst, heart rate, breathing, temperature, pain, and other visceral sensations. Interoception is processed primarily by the insula. In chronic pain, interoceptive awareness often becomes distorted, with the nervous system over-monitoring and misinterpreting normal bodily signals as threats.

L

Limbic System
A group of brain structures that process emotions, memory, motivation, and threat detection. Key structures include the amygdala, hippocampus, anterior cingulate cortex, and insula. The limbic system transforms sensation into suffering by adding emotional weight to pain signals. In chronic pain, the limbic system often becomes hyperactive, amplifying pain through fear, catastrophizing, and stress responses.

Long COVID
A condition where symptoms persist for weeks or months following acute COVID-19 infection. Common

symptoms include fatigue, brain fog, pain, breathlessness, and dysautonomia. Long COVID shares mechanisms with ME/CFS, including potential viral persistence, immune dysregulation, and central nervous system sensitization.

Lyme Disease (Chronic Lyme)
 A tick-borne illness caused by Borrelia bacteria. While acute Lyme responds to antibiotics, some patients develop persistent symptoms including pain, fatigue, and cognitive difficulties. Whether this represents ongoing infection, immune dysfunction, or central sensitization remains debated. The term "chronic Lyme" is controversial, but the suffering is real.

M

Maladaptive Neuroplasticity
 The central concept of this book. While neuroplasticity—the brain's ability to reorganize itself—is usually beneficial, it can also learn harmful patterns. Maladaptive neuroplasticity occurs when the nervous system becomes too good at producing pain, creating persistent pain circuits, altered body maps, and hypersensitivity even after tissue healing. This is

the common mechanism linking fibromyalgia, EDS, CRPS, and other chronic conditions discussed in this book.

Mast Cell Activation Syndrome (MCAS)
A condition where mast cells (immune cells that release histamine and other chemicals) become overactive, triggering allergic-type reactions without true allergies. Symptoms include flushing, hives, digestive problems, rapid heart rate, and pain. MCAS commonly co-occurs with EDS, POTS, and fibromyalgia, suggesting shared mechanisms of nervous system and immune dysregulation.

Mirror Therapy
A rehabilitation technique using mirrors to create the visual illusion of movement in a painful or missing limb. Originally developed for phantom limb pain, mirror therapy works through visual feedback to the brain, helping reorganize cortical maps. It has shown effectiveness in CRPS and other pain conditions involving cortical reorganization.

Myalgic Encephalomyelitis/Chronic Fatigue Syndrome (ME/CFS)
A complex condition characterized by severe, disabling fatigue not improved by rest, often worsened by physical or mental exertion (post-exertional malaise).

Also includes pain, cognitive difficulties, sleep disturbances, and dysautonomia. ME/CFS may involve viral triggers, immune dysfunction, mitochondrial problems, and central sensitization. It shares significant overlap with fibromyalgia and often co-occurs with EDS and POTS.

N

Neuroinflammation
Inflammation within the central nervous system, involving activation of glial cells and release of inflammatory chemicals. Research has found neuroinflammation in fibromyalgia, ME/CFS, and other chronic pain conditions. Unlike peripheral inflammation, neuroinflammation directly affects neural function and can contribute to pain amplification, fatigue, and cognitive difficulties.

Neuromatrix Theory
A theory proposed by Ronald Melzack suggesting that pain is not simply a response to sensory input but is generated by a network (matrix) of brain regions working together. The neuromatrix integrates sensory, emotional, and cognitive information to create the pain

experience. This theory explains why pain can exist without tissue damage and why psychological factors profoundly influence pain.

Neuropathic Pain

Pain caused by damage or disease affecting the nervous system itself (nerves, spinal cord, or brain). Neuropathic pain often feels like burning, shooting, stabbing, or electric shock-like sensations. Examples include diabetic neuropathy, post-herpetic neuralgia (shingles pain), and phantom limb pain. Neuropathic pain results from misfiring or damaged pain pathways.

Neuroplasticity

The brain and nervous system's ability to reorganize, form new connections, and change in response to experience. This capacity allows learning, recovery from injury, and adaptation. However, neuroplasticity can be maladaptive when the nervous system learns harmful patterns like chronic pain circuits. The good news: just as the nervous system learned pain, it can learn safety and pain reduction.

Nervous System Regulation

The process of shifting the nervous system away from chronic fight-or-flight toward a more balanced state with better access to parasympathetic "rest-and-digest" function. In practice, this includes breathwork, grounding, sleep support, gentle movement, connection, and trauma-informed therapies.

Nociception

The detection of potentially harmful stimuli by specialized sensory receptors (nociceptors). Nociception is the neurological process of sensing damage or threat—it's the signal, not the experience. You can have nociception without pain (under anesthesia) or pain without nociception (central sensitization). This distinction is crucial: pain is not just nociception, but the brain's interpretation of it.

Nociceptive Pain

Pain that arises from actual or threatened tissue damage, where nociceptors are working normally. This is "normal" pain—like a cut, burn, fracture, or sprained ankle. Nociceptive pain is protective, alerting you to harm and encouraging behaviors that promote healing. It typically resolves as tissues heal.

Nociceptors

Specialized sensory receptors that detect potentially harmful stimuli (mechanical, thermal, or chemical). When activated, nociceptors send signals to the spinal cord and brain, which may be interpreted as pain. However, nociceptor activation doesn't always produce pain—the signal must pass through multiple levels of processing and modulation.

Nociplastic Pain
A relatively new pain category (recognized by the International Association for the Study of Pain in 2017) describing pain that arises from altered pain processing despite no clear tissue damage or nerve lesion. Nociplastic pain results from changes in how the nervous system processes signals—essentially, a dysregulated pain system. Fibromyalgia is the prototypical nociplastic pain condition.

P

Pacing
A self-management strategy that involves breaking activities into smaller chunks with rest periods to avoid boom-bust cycles and post-exertional crashes. Effective pacing requires finding your sustainable baseline (what you can do consistently) and gradually building from there. It's not about avoiding activity—it's about managing energy and nervous system load strategically.

Pain Catastrophizing (See: Catastrophizing)

Pain Loop

A self-reinforcing cycle in which pain disrupts sleep, movement, and stress regulation; those disruptions then increase pain sensitivity, feeding back into more pain. Over time, the nervous system learns this loop as the default pattern. Much of the work in this book is about interrupting and retraining this loop.

Parasympathetic Nervous System

The division of the autonomic nervous system responsible for "rest and digest" functions. It slows heart rate, promotes digestion, and supports recovery and healing. In chronic pain, the parasympathetic system is often under-active, preventing the body from accessing restorative states. Interventions like breathwork, mindfulness, and vagal stimulation aim to activate this system.

Periaqueductal Gray (PAG)

A region in the midbrain that plays a key role in descending pain modulation. The PAG can trigger the release of endogenous opioids and activate inhibitory pathways that dampen pain signals coming up from the spinal cord. It's one of the brain's built-in "pain relief hubs."

Peripheral Nervous System

All the nerves outside the brain and spinal cord,

including sensory and motor nerves throughout the body. The peripheral nervous system detects stimuli and sends signals to the CNS. In chronic pain, both peripheral and central nervous system changes often occur together.

Phantom Limb Pain

Pain perceived in a limb that has been amputated. This phenomenon demonstrates that pain is generated by the brain, not just the body. Phantom limb pain results from cortical reorganization—the brain's map of the missing limb persists and can generate pain signals. Treatments like mirror therapy work by providing the brain with new visual information to reorganize these maps.

Placebo Effect

A genuine therapeutic effect produced by an inactive treatment, resulting from the person's expectations and beliefs. The placebo effect is real and measurable—it can trigger release of endogenous opioids, reduce pain, and improve function. This demonstrates the powerful role of expectation and belief in shaping pain perception. Using the placebo effect therapeutically (through education, positive framing, and therapeutic alliance) is not deception—it's harnessing the brain's natural pain-modulating abilities.

Post-Exertional Malaise (PEM)

A hallmark symptom of ME/CFS where even minor physical or cognitive exertion triggers a crash—severe worsening of fatigue, pain, cognitive difficulties, and other symptoms that can last days or weeks. PEM may result from mitochondrial dysfunction, immune activation, or nervous system dysregulation. Managing PEM requires careful pacing and energy conservation.

Postural Orthostatic Tachycardia Syndrome (POTS)

A form of dysautonomia where standing upright triggers an excessive increase in heart rate (typically 30+ beats per minute within 10 minutes of standing) without a significant drop in blood pressure. Symptoms include dizziness, lightheadedness, palpitations, fatigue, brain fog, and exercise intolerance. POTS commonly co-occurs with EDS, MCAS, and ME/CFS.

Post-Traumatic Stress Disorder (PTSD)

A condition that develops after experiencing or witnessing traumatic events. PTSD involves intrusive memories, hypervigilance, avoidance, and emotional dysregulation. Importantly for this book, PTSD frequently includes chronic pain—the trauma rewires both emotional circuits and pain processing systems. The body "keeps the score," holding trauma not just as memory but as physical sensation.

Predictive Coding

A theory of brain function proposing that the brain constantly generates predictions about incoming sensory information and compares these predictions with actual input. When predictions don't match reality, the brain updates its model. In chronic pain, faulty predictions can lead the brain to "fill in" pain signals that aren't there or amplify signals that are. Expectations powerfully shape experience through this mechanism.

Prefrontal Cortex

The front-most region of the brain, responsible for executive functions like decision-making, planning, attention, and emotional regulation. The prefrontal cortex interprets pain, assigns meaning to it, and determines how much attention to give it. Cognitive factors (catastrophizing, expectation, beliefs about pain) are processed here, profoundly influencing pain perception and behavior.

Proprioception

The sense of your body's position and movement in space. Proprioceptors in muscles, tendons, and joints send constant feedback to the brain about where your body parts are and what they're doing. In conditions like EDS, proprioceptive deficits are common—the brain receives unreliable information about joint position, requiring constant conscious correction and contributing to fatigue, clumsiness, and pain.

R

Referred Pain
Pain felt in a location different from the actual source. The classic example: a heart attack causing left arm pain. Referred pain occurs because of how nerve pathways converge in the spinal cord and how cortical body maps are organized. Pain from one region can "spill over" into neighboring regions on the cortical map, causing pain to be felt in areas without tissue damage.

Reframing
A cognitive technique where you consciously change how you interpret a situation. In pain management, reframing might mean shifting from "this pain means I'm broken" to "this is my nervous system on high alert—I can teach it to calm down." Reframing doesn't deny pain—it changes the emotional and cognitive weight attached to it, which can reduce limbic amplification.

REM Sleep (Rapid Eye Movement Sleep)
The sleep stage associated with dreaming, emotional processing, and memory consolidation. REM sleep helps integrate new learning, including nervous-system retraining from movement and exposure work. Fragmented REM sleep can worsen mood, emotional resilience, and the brain's ability to encode new patterns.

S

Sensitization (See: Central Sensitization)

Sensory Overload / Sensory Load
A state where the nervous system is flooded with more input than it can process—noise, lights, screens, complex environments, emotional demands, and internal sensations. In a sensitized nervous system, this overload makes pain and other symptoms feel more intense and more intrusive, even without new injury.

Sleep Apnea
A sleep disorder where breathing repeatedly stops and starts during sleep, usually due to airway collapse. It fragments deep and REM sleep, lowers oxygen levels,

and significantly worsens pain sensitivity, fatigue, and cognitive function. CPAP (continuous positive airway pressure) is a common treatment.

Sleep Architecture

The overall structure and pattern of sleep across the night—the sequence and proportion of N1, N2, deep (N3) sleep, and REM. Chronic pain often disrupts sleep architecture, reducing deep and REM sleep and leaving people stuck in lighter stages. That disruption prevents the nervous system from completing its nightly "reset."

Sleep Hygiene

Practices and environmental conditions that promote quality sleep. These include consistent sleep/wake times, a dark and cool bedroom, limiting screen time before bed, avoiding caffeine and heavy meals close to bedtime, and creating a calming bedtime routine. In chronic pain, sleep hygiene is crucial because poor sleep worsens pain, and pain disrupts sleep—creating a vicious cycle.

Somatosensory Cortex

The brain region that processes sensory information from the body, including touch, temperature, pain, and body position. The somatosensory cortex contains organized maps of the body (cortical body maps), with adjacent body regions represented in adjacent brain areas. These maps are plastic—they reorganize based on experience, injury, and use. In chronic pain, these maps often become distorted.

Stress Hormones

Hormones released in response to stress, mainly cortisol and adrenaline (epinephrine). Short-term, they help you handle threats. When stress hormones stay elevated, they disrupt sleep, keep the body in fight-or-flight, and lower pain thresholds.

Stress Response

The body's reaction to perceived threat, involving activation of the hypothalamic-pituitary-adrenal (HPA) axis and sympathetic nervous system. This triggers release of stress hormones (cortisol, adrenaline), increases heart rate and blood pressure, tenses muscles, and suppresses non-essential functions. Acute stress responses are protective, but chronic activation contributes to pain, fatigue, immune dysfunction, and other health problems.

Sympathetic Nervous System

The division of the autonomic nervous system responsible for activating the body during stress—the "fight-or-flight" response. When activated, it increases heart rate, blood pressure, and muscle tension while suppressing digestion and healing. In chronic pain, the sympathetic system often stays chronically activated, preventing recovery and amplifying pain signals.

Syndrome Overlap
The pattern where multiple chronic conditions frequently occur together in the same person. Examples: fibromyalgia with EDS, POTS with MCAS, ME/CFS with PTSD. Rather than bad luck, syndrome overlap suggests shared underlying mechanisms—particularly nervous system dysregulation and maladaptive neuroplasticity. Understanding this helps explain why treating one condition often helps others.

T

Thalamus
A brain structure that acts as a relay station for sensory information, routing signals to appropriate regions of the cortex. Almost all sensory input (except smell) passes through the thalamus. In chronic pain, thalamic function can become altered, contributing to pain amplification and processing abnormalities.

Trauma

Experiences that overwhelm a person's ability to cope, often involving threat to physical or psychological safety. Trauma doesn't require physical injury—emotional trauma is equally real and impactful. Trauma rewires the nervous system, affecting threat detection, emotional regulation, pain processing, and stress responses. "The body keeps the score"—trauma is held not just in memory but in physical patterns of tension, pain, and dysregulation.

Trigger Point

A hyperirritable spot in muscle that produces pain, often referring pain to other areas. Traditional models viewed trigger points as purely muscular phenomena. This book proposes that many trigger point patterns reflect cortical reorganization—the brain's remapped body representation causing pain to "spread" across neighboring regions on the cortical map, regardless of peripheral tissue state.

V

Vagus Nerve

The longest cranial nerve, running from the brainstem

through the neck, chest, and abdomen. The vagus nerve is the primary nerve of the parasympathetic nervous system. Vagal tone (how well the vagus nerve functions) influences heart rate variability, inflammation, digestion, and emotional regulation. Low vagal tone is common in chronic pain and trauma. Vagal stimulation techniques (breathing exercises, cold exposure, singing, humming) can help activate the parasympathetic system and reduce pain.

W

Wide Dynamic Range (WDR) Neurons
Nerve cells in the spinal cord that respond to both non-painful and painful stimuli. WDR neurons can be "wound up" with repeated stimulation, becoming more excitable and contributing to central sensitization. These neurons are key players in the transition from acute to chronic pain.

Wind-Up
A phenomenon where repeated pain signals to the spinal cord cause progressively stronger responses in spinal neurons. Like a crescendo that never stops, wind-up makes the nervous system increasingly

responsive to pain. This process contributes to central sensitization and explains why repeated painful experiences can make the nervous system more sensitive over time.

4–7–8 Breathing

A specific breathing pattern used to calm the nervous system: inhale through the nose for a count of 4, hold for a count of 7, then exhale slowly through the mouth for a count of 8. Repeating this several times can reduce arousal, slow heart rate, and nudge the system toward parasympathetic dominance.

Notes on Usage

This glossary defines terms as they are used within the context of this book. Some terms may have broader or more specific meanings in other contexts. When in doubt about how a term is being used, refer back to the relevant chapter for fuller explanation.

You don't need to memorize every term—use this glossary as a reference when you encounter unfamiliar words. Nearly every term points back to the same underlying mechanisms: how the nervous system learns, adapts, and sometimes gets stuck in harmful patterns. Whether we're talking about central sensitization, cortical reorganization, limbic amplification, or autonomic dysregulation—these are all expressions of maladaptive neuroplasticity. Understanding that unifying thread helps make sense of why so many conditions cluster together and why similar interventions help across different diagnoses.

Recommended Reading

This book is a lens, not a comprehensive encyclopedia. Each condition and intervention discussed here has depth and nuance that goes beyond what we can cover in a single volume. Below are resources I recommend for readers who want to go deeper into the science, the lived experience, and the practical application of these concepts.

Fibromyalgia

- Liptan, G. (2016). *The FibroManual: A Complete Fibromyalgia Treatment Guide for You and Your Doctor.* Ballantine Books.

- Starlanyl, D., & Copeland, M. E. (2001). *Fibromyalgia & Chronic Myofascial Pain: A Survival Manual* (2nd ed.). New Harbinger Publications.

Ehlers-Danlos Syndrome

- Russek, L., & Hennessey, E. (Eds.). (2020). *Disjointed: Navigating the Diagnosis and Management of Hypermobile Ehlers-Danlos Syndrome and Hypermobility Spectrum Disorders.* Independently published.

- Knight, I. (2020). *A Guide to Living with Ehlers-Danlos Syndrome (Hypermobility Type).* Singing Dragon.

CRPS (Complex Regional Pain Syndrome)

- Moseley, G. L., & Butler, D. S. (2017). *Explain Pain Supercharged.* NOI Group.

- Harden, R. N., et al. (Eds.). (2013). *Complex Regional Pain Syndrome: Treatment Guidelines.* Millet Publishing.

PTSD & Trauma

- van der Kolk, B. (2014). *The Body Keeps the Score: Brain, Mind, and Body in the Healing of Trauma.* Viking.

- Levine, P. A. (2010). *In an Unspoken Voice: How the Body Releases Trauma and Restores Goodness.* North Atlantic Books.

- Maté, G. (2003). *When the Body Says No: Exploring the Stress-Disease Connection.* Wiley.

Pain Science (General)

- Moseley, G. L., & Butler, D. S. (2013). *Explain Pain* (2nd ed.). NOI Group.
- Louw, A. (2013). *Why Do I Hurt? A Patient Book about the Neuroscience of Pain.* OPTP.
- Gordon, A. (2021). *The Way Out: A Revolutionary, Scientifically Proven Approach to Healing Chronic Pain.* Avery.
- Schubiner, H. (2010). *Unlearn Your Pain: A 28-Day Process to Reprogram Your Brain.* Mind Body Publishing.

Chronic Illness & Patient Perspective

- O'Rourke, M. (2022). *The Invisible Kingdom: Reimagining Chronic Illness.* Riverhead Books.

Neuroplasticity, Mental Health & the Brain

- Doidge, N. (2007). *The Brain That Changes Itself: Stories of Personal Triumph from the Frontiers of Brain Science.* Viking.
  - Essential reading on neuroplasticity in action, including how the brain rewires itself in response to pain, trauma, and recovery.

- Doidge, N. (2015). *The Brain's Way of Healing: Remarkable Discoveries and Recoveries from the Frontiers of Neuroplasticity.* Viking.
  - Explores non-pharmaceutical approaches to healing chronic pain and neurological conditions through neuroplastic mechanisms.

- Schwartz, J. M., & Begley, S. (2002). *The Mind and the Brain: Neuroplasticity and the Power of Mental Force.* ReganBooks/HarperCollins.
  - Demonstrates how mental practices can reshape brain circuitry, with applications to OCD, anxiety, and depression.

- Arden, J. B. (2010). *Rewire Your Brain: Think Your Way to a Better Life.* Wiley.

- Practical guide to using neuroplasticity principles to address anxiety, depression, and negative thought patterns.

Movement & Exercise

- Cook, G. (2010). *Movement: Functional Movement Systems.* On Target Publications.
- McGill, S. (2015). *Back Mechanic: The Step-by-Step McGill Method to Fix Back Pain.* Backfitpro Inc.

Nutrition (Evidence-Based)

- Schoenfeld, B. J., & Contreras, B. (2020). *The Science of Nutrition.* Human Kinetics.
- Greger, M. (2015). *How Not to Die: Discover the Foods Scientifically Proven to Prevent and Reverse Disease.* Flatiron Books.

Mindfulness & Nervous System Regulation

- Kabat-Zinn, J. (2013). *Full Catastrophe Living: Using the Wisdom of Your Body and Mind to Face Stress, Pain, and Illness* (Revised ed.). Bantam.

- Dana, D. (2018). *The Polyvagal Theory in Therapy: Engaging the Rhythm of Regulation.* W. W. Norton & Company.

- Porges, S. W. (2011). *The Polyvagal Theory: Neurophysiological Foundations of Emotions, Attachment, Communication, and Self-Regulation.* W. W. Norton & Company.

  - Foundational text on the vagus nerve, autonomic regulation, and how safety signals calm the nervous system.

Manual Therapy & Bodywork

- Myers, T. W. (2014). *Anatomy Trains: Myofascial Meridians for Manual and Movement Therapists* (3rd ed.). Churchill Livingstone.

- Travell, J. G., & Simons, D. G. (1999). *Myofascial Pain and Dysfunction: The Trigger Point Manual* (2nd ed.). Lippincott Williams & Wilkins.

Understanding Depression & Anxiety Through a Neuroplastic Lens

While this book focuses on chronic pain conditions, the mechanisms of maladaptive neuroplasticity also help explain how anxiety and depression can become "learned" states in the brain. These books explore that connection:

- **Yapko, M. D. (2009).** *Depression Is Contagious: How the Most Common Mood Disorder Is Spreading Around the World and How to Stop It.* Free Press.
  o Examines how depression can be understood as learned helplessness and cognitive patterns that become neurologically reinforced.

- **Schwartz, J. M., & Gladding, R. (2011).** *You Are Not Your Brain: The 4-Step Solution for Changing Bad Habits, Ending Unhealthy Thinking, and Taking Control of Your Life.* Avery.
  o Shows how the brain's circuitry can be reshaped to break cycles of anxiety, depression, and compulsive thinking.

- **Hanson, R. (2013).** *Hardwiring Happiness: The New Brain Science of Contentment, Calm, and Confidence.* Harmony.

    o   Practical guide to using neuroplasticity to overcome negative thought patterns and build resilience against anxiety and depression.

- **Begley, S. (2007).** *Train Your Mind, Change Your Brain: How a New Science Reveals Our Extraordinary Potential to Transform Ourselves.* Ballantine Books.

    o   Explores how meditation, cognitive training, and mindfulness can reshape the brain's response to stress, anxiety, and depression.

This reading list is not exhaustive, but it represents some of the best resources I know for going deeper into the topics we've touched on. Use them as starting points for your own exploration.

Master Bibliography

Abbasi, B., Kimiagar, M., Sadeghniiat, K., Shirazi, M. M., Hedayati, M., & Rashidkhani, B. (2012). The effect of magnesium supplementation on primary insomnia in elderly: A double-blind placebo-controlled clinical trial. *Journal of Research in Medical Sciences*, 17(12), 1161–1169.

Afari, N., Ahumada, S. M., Wright, L. J., Mostoufi, S., Golnari, G., Reis, V., & Cuneo, J. G. (2014). Psychological trauma and functional somatic syndromes: A systematic review and meta-analysis. *Psychosomatic Medicine*, 76(1), 2–11.

Albrecht, D. S., Forsberg, A., Sandström, A., et al. (2019). Brain glial activation in fibromyalgia: A multi-site positron emission tomography investigation. *Brain, Behavior, and Immunity*, 75, 72–83.

Anderson, L. K., & Lane, K. R. (2021). The diagnostic journey in adults with hypermobile Ehlers-Danlos syndrome and hypermobility spectrum disorders. *Journal of the American Association of Nurse Practitioners*, 34(4), 639–648.

Antcliff, D., Keeley, P., Campbell, M., Oldham, J., & Woby, S. (2013). Activity pacing: Moving beyond the controversy to principles and practice. *Clinical Rehabilitation*, 27(12), 1099–1107.

Apkarian, A. V., Baliki, M. N., & Farmer, M. A. (2013). Predicting transition to chronic pain. *Current Opinion in Neurology*, 26(4), 360–367.

Apkarian, A. V., Baliki, M. N., & Geha, P. Y. (2009). Towards a theory of chronic pain. *Progress in Neurobiology*, 87(2), 81–97.

Apkarian, A. V., Bushnell, M. C., Treede, R. D., & Zubieta, J. K. (2005). Human brain mechanisms of pain perception and regulation in health and disease. *European Journal of Pain*, 9(4), 463–484.

Baeza-Velasco, C., Gély-Nargeot, M. C., & Bulbena, A. (2018). Joint hypermobility, anxiety, and psychosomatic symptoms: The link and the role of autonomic hyperarousal. *Journal of Psychosomatic Research*, 111, 77–82.

Baliki, M. N., et al. (2012). Corticostriatal functional connectivity predicts transition to chronic back pain. *Nature Neuroscience*, 15(8), 1117–1119.

Bandura, A. (1997). *Self-efficacy: The exercise of control*. W.H. Freeman and Company.

Bannai, M., & Kawai, N. (2012). New therapeutic strategy for amino acid medicine: Glycine improves the quality of sleep. *Journal of Pharmacological Sciences*, 118(2), 145–148.

Barnden, L. R., Crouch, B., Kwiatek, R., Burnet, R., Del Fante, P., & MacKay, C. (2011). A brain MRI study of chronic fatigue syndrome: Evidence of brainstem dysfunction and altered autonomic regulation. *NMR in Biomedicine*, 24(10), 1302–1311.

Basbaum, A. I., Bautista, D. M., Scherrer, G., & Julius, D. (2009). Cellular and molecular mechanisms of pain. *Cell*, 139(2), 267–284.

Basbaum, A. I., & Fields, H. L. (1984). Endogenous pain control systems: Brainstem spinal pathways and endorphin circuitry. *Annual Review of Neuroscience*, 7, 309–338.

Bathen, T., Hångmann, A. B., Hoff, M., Andersen, L. Ø., & Rand-Hendriksen, S. (2013). Multidisciplinary treatment of disability in Ehlers-Danlos syndrome hypermobility type/hypermobility syndrome: A pilot study using a combination of physical and cognitive-behavioral therapy on 12 women. *American Journal of Medical Genetics Part A*, 161(12), 3005–3011.

Baumeister, R. F., & Leary, M. R. (1995). The need to belong: Desire for interpersonal attachments as a fundamental human motivation. *Psychological Bulletin*, 117(3), 497–529.

Benarroch, E. E. (2012). Postural tachycardia syndrome: A heterogeneous and multifactorial disorder. *Mayo Clinic Proceedings*, 87(12), 1214–1225.

Bernardy, K., Klose, P., Busch, A. J., Choy, E. H., & Häuser, W. (2013). Cognitive behavioural therapies for fibromyalgia. *Cochrane Database of Systematic Reviews*, 9, CD009796.

Bialosky, J. E., Bishop, M. D., Price, D. D., Robinson, M. E., & George, S. Z. (2009). The mechanisms of manual therapy in the treatment of musculoskeletal pain: A comprehensive model. *Manual Therapy*, 14(5), 531–538.

Bialosky, J. E., et al. (2009). Placebo response to manual therapy: Something out of nothing? *Journal of Manual & Manipulative Therapy*, 17(1), 11–18.

Birbaumer, N., Lutzenberger, W., Montoya, P., Larbig, W., Unertl, K., Töpfner, S., Grodd, W., Taub, E., & Flor, H. (1997). Effects of regional anesthesia on phantom limb pain are mirrored in changes in cortical reorganization. *Journal of Neuroscience*, 17(14), 5503–5508.

Birklein, F., & Schlereth, T. (2015). Complex regional pain syndrome—significant progress in understanding. *Pain*, 156(Suppl 1), S94–S103.

Booth, J., Moseley, G. L., Schiltenwolf, M., Cashin, A., Davies, M., & Hübscher, M. (2017). Exercise for chronic musculoskeletal pain: A biopsychosocial approach. *Musculoskeletal Care*, 15(4), 413–421.

Born, J., Hansen, K., Marshall, L., Mölle, M., & Fehm, H. L. (1999). Timing the end of nocturnal sleep. *Nature*, 397(6714), 29–30.

Born, J., Lange, T., Hansen, K., Mölle, M., & Fehm, H. L. (1997). Effects of sleep and circadian rhythm on human circulating immune cells. *Journal of Immunology*, 158(9), 4454–4464.

Borsook, D., Maleki, N., Becerra, L., & McEwen, B. (2012). Understanding migraine through the lens of maladaptive stress responses: A model disease of allostatic load. *Neuron*, 73(2), 219–234.

Bowering, K. J., et al. (2013). The effects of graded motor imagery and its components on chronic pain: A systematic review and meta-analysis. *The Journal of Pain*, 14(1), 3–13.

Brown, B. (2012). *Daring Greatly: How the Courage to Be Vulnerable Transforms the Way We Live, Love, Parent, and Lead*. Gotham Books.

Brown, C. A., & Jones, A. K. P. (2010). Meditation experience predicts less negative appraisal of pain: Electrophysiological support for the mindfulness–stress buffering account. *Pain*, 150(3), 428–439.

Büchel, C., Geuter, S., Sprenger, C., & Eippert, F. (2014). Placebo analgesia: A predictive coding perspective. *Neuron*, 81(6), 1223–1239.

Busch, A. J., Webber, S. C., Richards, R. S., et al. (2013). Resistance exercise training for fibromyalgia. *Cochrane Database of Systematic Reviews*, 12, CD010884.

Bushnell, M. C., Ceko, M., & Low, L. A. (2013). Cognitive and emotional control of pain and its disruption in chronic pain. *Nature Reviews Neuroscience*, 14(7), 502–511.

Bushnell, M. C., Čeko, M., & Low, L. A. (2013). Cognitive and emotional control of pain and its disruption in chronic pain. *Nature Reviews Neuroscience*, 14(7), 502–511.

Butler, D. S., & Moseley, G. L. (2013). *Explain Pain* (2nd ed.). Noigroup Publications.

Campbell, L. F. (1982). Diving reflex in man: Its relation to isometric and dynamic exercise. *Journal of Applied Physiology*, 52(1), 115–119.

Cano, A., & Williams, A. C. (2010). Social interaction in pain: Reinforcing pain behaviors or building intimacy? *Pain*, 149(1), 9–11.

Castori, M., Morlino, S., Celletti, C., Ghibellini, G., Bruschini, M., Grammatico, P., ... & Camerota, F. (2013). Re-writing the natural history of pain and related symptoms in the joint hypermobility syndrome/Ehlers-Danlos syndrome, hypermobility type. *American Journal of Medical Genetics Part A*, 161(12), 2989–3004.

Charmaz, K. (1983). Loss of self: A fundamental form of suffering in the chronically ill. *Sociology of Health & Illness*, 5(2), 168–195.

Clauw, D. J. (2014). Fibromyalgia: A clinical review. *JAMA*, 311(15), 1547–1555.

Clauw, D. J. (2015). Diagnosing and treating chronic musculoskeletal pain based on the underlying mechanism(s). *Best Practice & Research Clinical Rheumatology*, 29(1), 6–19.

Clear, J. (2018). *Atomic Habits: An Easy & Proven Way to Build Good Habits & Break Bad Ones*. Avery.

Coan, J. A., & Sbarra, D. A. (2015). Social baseline theory: The social regulation of risk and effort. *Current Opinion in Psychology*, 1, 87–91.

Cook, D. B., Lange, G., Ciccone, D. S., Liu, W. C., Steffener, J., & Natelson, B. H. (2004). Functional imaging of pain in patients with primary fibromyalgia. *Journal of Rheumatology*, 31(2), 364–378.

Cormier, S., Lavigne, G. L., Choinière, M., & Rainville, P. (2016). Expectations predict chronic pain treatment outcomes. *Pain*, 157(2), 329–338.

Costigan, M., Scholz, J., & Woolf, C. J. (2009). Neuropathic pain: A maladaptive response of the nervous system to damage. *Annual Review of Neuroscience*, 32, 1–32.

Craig, A. D. (2002). How do you feel? Interoception: The sense of the physiological condition of the body. *Nature Reviews Neuroscience*, 3(8), 655–666.

Craig, A. D. (2003). Interoception: The sense of the physiological condition of the body. *Current Opinion in Neurobiology*, 13(4), 500–505.

Craig, A. D. (2009). How do you feel now? The anterior insula and human awareness. *Nature Reviews Neuroscience*, 10(1), 59–70.

Critchley, H. D., Wiens, S., Rotshtein, P., Öhman, A., & Dolan, R. J. (2004). Neural systems supporting interoceptive awareness. *Nature Neuroscience*, 7(2), 189–195.

Crombez, G., Eccleston, C., Van Damme, S., Vlaeyen, J. W., & Karoly, P. (2012). Fear-avoidance model of chronic pain: The next generation. *The Clinical Journal of Pain*, 28(6), 475–483.

Dahl, J., Wilson, K. G., & Nilsson, A. (2004). Acceptance and commitment therapy and the treatment of persons at risk for long-term disability resulting from stress and pain symptoms: A preliminary randomized trial. *Behavior Therapy*, 35(4), 785–801.

Dahlhamer, J., Lucas, J., Zelaya, C., et al. (2018). Prevalence of chronic pain and high-impact chronic pain among adults — United States, 2016. *Morbidity and Mortality Weekly Report*, 67(36), 1001–1006.

De Wandele, I., Rombaut, L., Leybaert, L., Van de Borne, P., De Backer, T., Malfait, F., ... & Calders, P. (2014). Dysautonomia and its underlying mechanisms in the hypermobility type of Ehlers-Danlos syndrome. *Seminars in Arthritis and Rheumatism*, 44(1), 93–100.

Diatchenko, L., et al. (2013). The phenotypic and genetic signatures of common musculoskeletal pain conditions. *Nature Reviews Rheumatology*, 9(6), 340–350.

Di Lernia, D., Serino, S., & Riva, G. (2016). Pain in the body. Altered interoception in chronic pain conditions: A systematic review. *Neuroscience & Biobehavioral Reviews*, 71, 328–341.

Doidge, N. (2007). *The Brain That Changes Itself: Stories of Personal Triumph from the Frontiers of Brain Science*. Penguin Books.

Doubell, T. P., Mannion, R. J., & Woolf, C. J. (1999). The dorsal horn: State-dependent sensory processing, plasticity, and the generation of pain. In *Textbook of Pain* (4th ed., pp. 165–181). Churchill Livingstone.

Dupuy, E. G., Leconte, P., Vlamynck, E., Sultan, A., Chesneau, C., Denise, P., ... & Decker, L. M. (2017). Ehlers-Danlos Syndrome, Hypermobility Type: Impact of Somatosensory Orthoses on Postural Control (A Pilot Study). *Frontiers in Human Neuroscience*, 11, 283.

Eccleston, C., & Crombez, G. (2007). Worry and chronic pain: A misdirected problem solving model. *Pain*, 132(3), 233–236.

Edwards, R. R., Dworkin, R. H., Sullivan, M. D., Turk, D. C., & Wasan, A. D. (2016). The role of psychosocial processes in the development and maintenance of chronic pain. *The Journal of Pain*, 17(9), T70–T92.

Eisenberger, N. I. (2012). Broken hearts and broken bones: A neural perspective on the similarities between social and physical pain. *Current Directions in Psychological Science*, 21(1), 42–47.

Eisenberger, N. I., & Cole, S. W. (2012). Social neuroscience and health: Neurophysiological mechanisms linking social ties with physical health. *Nature Neuroscience*, 15(5), 669–674.

Eisenberger, N. I., Lieberman, M. D., & Williams, K. D. (2003). Does rejection hurt? An fMRI study of social exclusion. *Science*, 302(5643), 290–292.

Emmons, R. A., & McCullough, M. E. (2003). Counting blessings versus burdens: An experimental investigation of gratitude and subjective well-being in daily life. *Journal of Personality and Social Psychology*, 84(2), 377–389.

Fairweather, D., Bruno, K. A., Darakjian, A. A., Bruce, B. K., Gehin, J. M., Kotha, A., Jain, A., Peng, Z., Hodge, D. O., Rozen, T. D., Munipalli, B., Rivera, F. A., Malavet, P. A., & Knight, D. R. T. (2023). High overlap in patients diagnosed with hypermobile Ehlers-Danlos syndrome or hypermobility spectrum disorders with fibromyalgia and 40 self-reported symptoms and comorbidities. *Frontiers in Medicine*, 10, 1096180.

Felitti, V. J., Anda, R. F., Nordenberg, D., Williamson, D. F., Spitz, A. M., Edwards, V., Koss, M. P., & Marks, J. S. (1998). Relationship of childhood abuse and household dysfunction to many of the leading causes of death in adults: The Adverse Childhood Experiences (ACE) Study. *American Journal of Preventive Medicine*, 14(4), 245–258.

Ferrell, W. R., Tennant, N., Sturrock, R. D., Ashton, L., Creed, G., Brydson, G., & Rafferty, D. (2004). Amelioration of symptoms by enhancement of proprioception in patients with joint hypermobility syndrome. *Arthritis & Rheumatism*, 50(10), 3323–3328.

Field, T. (2016). Massage therapy research review. *Complementary Therapies in Clinical Practice*, 24, 19–31.

Fields, H. L. (2004). State-dependent opioid control of pain. *Nature Reviews Neuroscience*, 5(7), 565–575.

Finan, P. H., Goodin, B. R., & Smith, M. T. (2013). The association of sleep and pain: An update and a path forward. *The Journal of Pain*, 14(12), 1539–1552.

Flor, H. (2003). Cortical reorganisation and chronic pain: Implications for rehabilitation. *Journal of Rehabilitation Medicine*, 41(Suppl.), 66–72.

Flor, H. (2012). New developments in the understanding and management of persistent pain. *Current Opinion in Psychiatry*, 25(2), 109–113.

Flor, H., Braun, C., Elbert, T., & Birbaumer, N. (1997). Extensive reorganization of primary somatosensory cortex in chronic back pain patients. *Neuroscience Letters*, 224(1), 5–8.

Flor, H., Elbert, T., Knecht, S., et al. (1995). Phantom-limb pain as a perceptual correlate of cortical reorganization following arm amputation. *Nature*, 375, 482–484.

Flor, H., Elbert, T., Knecht, S., Wienbruch, C., Pantev, C., Birbaumer, N., Larbig, W., & Taub, E. (1995). Phantom-limb pain as a perceptual correlate of cortical reorganization following arm amputation. *Nature*, 375(6531), 482–484.

Foa, E. B., et al. (2007). Randomized trial of prolonged exposure for posttraumatic stress disorder with and without cognitive restructuring. *Journal of Consulting and Clinical Psychology*, 75(6), 904–913.

Fuentes, J., et al. (2014). Enhanced therapeutic alliance modulates pain intensity and muscle pain sensitivity in patients with chronic low back pain: An experimental controlled study. *Physical Therapy*, 94(4), 477–489.

Furlan, A. D., Yazdi, F., Tsertsvadze, A., Gross, A., Van Tulder, M., Santaguida, L., Gagnier, J., Ammendolia, C., Dryden, T., & Doucette, S. (2010). A systematic review and meta-analysis of efficacy, cost-effectiveness, and safety of selected complementary and alternative medicine for neck and low-back pain. *Evidence-Based Complementary and Alternative Medicine*, 7(1), 95–113.

Gatchel, R. J., Peng, Y. B., Peters, M. L., Fuchs, P. N., & Turk, D. C. (2007). The biopsychosocial approach to chronic pain: Scientific advances and future directions. *Psychological Bulletin*, 133(4), 581–624.

Geisser, M. E., Glass, J. M., Rajcevska, L. D., et al. (2008). A psychophysical study of auditory and pressure sensitivity in patients with fibromyalgia and healthy controls. *Journal of Pain*, 9(5), 417–422.

Geneen, L. J., Moore, R. A., Clarke, C., Martin, D., Colvin, L. A., & Smith, B. H. (2017). Physical activity and exercise for chronic pain in adults: An overview of Cochrane Reviews. *Cochrane Database of Systematic Reviews*, 4, CD011279.

Giamberardino, M. A., Affaitati, G., Fabrizio, A., & Costantini, R. (2011). Myofascial pain syndromes and their evaluation. *Best Practice & Research Clinical Rheumatology*, 25(2), 185–198.

Glass, J. M. (2009). Review of cognitive dysfunction in fibromyalgia: A convergence on working memory and attentional control impairments. *Rheumatic Disease Clinics of North America*, 35(2), 299–311.

Glans, M., Humble, M. B., Elwin, M., & Bejerot, S. (2024). Neuropsychological function and the relationship between subjective cognition, objective cognition, and symptoms in hypermobile Ehlers–Danlos syndrome. *APMR Reports*, 4(3), 100045.

Goessl, V. C., Curtiss, J. E., & Hofmann, S. G. (2017). The effect of heart rate variability biofeedback training on stress and anxiety: A meta-analysis. *Psychological Medicine*, 47(15), 2578–2586.

Haack, M., Simpson, N., Sethna, N., Kaur, S., & Mullington, J. (2020). Sleep deficiency and chronic pain: Potential underlying mechanisms and clinical implications. *Neuropsychopharmacology*, 45(1), 205–216.

Hall, A. M., et al. (2016). The effectiveness of Tai Chi for chronic musculoskeletal pain conditions: A systematic review and meta-analysis. *Arthritis & Rheumatology*, 69(9), 1876–1886.

Hannibal, K. E., & Bishop, M. D. (2014). Chronic stress, cortisol dysfunction, and pain: A psychoneuroendocrine rationale for stress management in pain rehabilitation. *Physical Therapy*, 94(12), 1816–1825.

Hansen, N., Kass-Iliyya, L., Namer, B., Saffer, D., Lampert, A., & Faber, C. G. (2019). Central sensitization in Ehlers-Danlos syndromes: An overlooked complication with consequences. *European Journal of Pain*, 23(7), 1199–1206.

Harden, R. N., et al. (2013). Complex regional pain syndrome: Practical diagnostic and treatment guidelines. *Pain Medicine*, 14(2), 180–229.

Harrison, F., & McLaughlin, K. A. (2019). Cognitive mechanisms of psychotherapy: Prediction, learning, and trust in the therapeutic process. *Current Opinion in Psychology*, 30, 44–49.

Häuser, W., Kosseva, M., Üceyler, N., Klose, P., & Sommer, C. (2011). Emotional, physical, and sexual abuse in fibromyalgia syndrome: A systematic review with meta-analysis. *Arthritis Care & Research*, 63(6), 808–820.

Hayes, J. P., et al. (2012). Quantitative meta-analysis of neural activity in posttraumatic stress disorder. *Biology of Mood & Anxiety Disorders*, 2, 9.

Herrero, J. F., Laird, J. M., & López-García, J. A. (2000). Wind-up of spinal cord neurones and pain sensation: Much ado about something? *Progress in Neurobiology*, 61(2), 169–203.

Hotamisligil, G. S. (2006). Inflammation and metabolic disorders. *Nature*, 444(7121), 860–867.

Hou, C. R., et al. (2002). Immediate effects of various physical therapeutic modalities on cervical myofascial pain and trigger-point sensitivity. *Archives of Physical Medicine and Rehabilitation*, 83(10), 1406–1414.

Hughes, L. S., Clark, J., Colclough, J. A., Dale, E., & McMillan, D. (2017). Acceptance and Commitment Therapy (ACT) for chronic pain: A systematic review and meta-analyses. *The Clinical Journal of Pain*, 33(6), 552–568.

Ibrahim, M. M., Shelbourne, K. D., & Freeman, J. W. (2012). Proprioception deficits in patients with joint hypermobility syndrome. *Clinical Orthopaedics and Related Research*, 470(10), 2889–2897.

Iliff, J. J., et al. (2012). A paravascular pathway facilitates CSF flow through the brain parenchyma and the clearance of interstitial solutes, including amyloid β. *Science Translational Medicine*, 4(147), 147ra111.

Jackson, T., Wang, Y., Wang, Y., & Fan, H. (2014). Self-efficacy and chronic pain outcomes: A meta-analytic review. *The Journal of Pain*, 15(8), 800–814.

Jensen, K. B., Loitoile, R., Kosek, E., et al. (2012). Patients with fibromyalgia display less functional connectivity in the brain's pain inhibitory network. *Pain*, 153(5), 1018–1026.

Jerath, R., Edry, J. W., Barnes, V. A., & Jerath, V. (2006). Physiology of long pranayamic breathing: Neural respiratory elements may provide a mechanism that explains how slow deep breathing shifts the autonomic nervous system. *Medical Hypotheses*, 67(3), 566–571.

Ji, R. R., Berta, T., & Nedergaard, M. (2013). Glia and pain: Is chronic pain a gliopathy? *Pain*, 154(Suppl 1), S10–S28.

Job Accommodation Network (JAN). (2021). *Accommodation and Compliance Series: Employees with Chronic Pain*. U.S. Department of Labor, Office of Disability Employment Policy.

Johnson, M. I., Paley, C. A., Howe, T. E., & Sluka, K. A. (2015). Transcutaneous electrical nerve stimulation for acute pain. *Cochrane Database of Systematic Reviews*, 6, CD006142.

Julien, N., Goffaux, P., Arsenault, P., & Marchand, S. (2005). Widespread pain in fibromyalgia is related to a deficit of endogenous pain inhibition. *Pain*, 114(1–2), 295–302.

Kabat-Zinn, J. (2013). *Full Catastrophe Living: Using the Wisdom of Your Body and Mind to Face Stress, Pain, and Illness* (Revised edition). Bantam.

Kamper, S. J., Apeldoorn, A. T., Chiarotto, A., et al. (2015). Multidisciplinary biopsychosocial rehabilitation for chronic low back pain. *Cochrane Database of Systematic Reviews*, (9), CD000963.

Khoury, B., Sharma, M., Rush, S. E., & Fournier, C. (2015). Mindfulness-based stress reduction for healthy individuals: A meta-analysis. *Journal of Psychosomatic Research*, 78(6), 519–528.

Kim, J., Loggia, M. L., Cahalan, C. M., et al. (2015). The somatosensory link in fibromyalgia: Functional connectivity of the primary somatosensory cortex is altered by sustained pain and is associated with clinical/autonomic dysfunction. *Arthritis & Rheumatology*, 67(5), 1395–1405.

Koenig, J., Jarczok, M. N., Ellis, R. J., Hillecke, T. K., & Thayer, J. F. (2014). Heart rate variability and experimentally induced pain in healthy adults: A systematic review. *European Journal of Pain*, 18(3), 301–314.

Kozlowska, K., Walker, P., McLean, L., & Carrive, P. (2015). Fear and the defense cascade: Clinical implications and management. *Harvard Review of Psychiatry*, 23(4), 263–287.

Lakhan, S. E., & Schofield, K. L. (2013). Mindfulness-based therapies in the treatment of somatization disorders: A systematic review and meta-analysis. *PLOS ONE*, 8(8), e71834.

Lassiter, D. G., et al. (2012). Counterregulatory responses to hypoglycemia. *Diabetes Care*, 35(6), 1380–1386.

Latremoliere, A., & Woolf, C. J. (2009). Central sensitization: A generator of pain hypersensitivity by central neural plasticity. *Journal of Pain*, 10(9), 895–926.

LeDoux, J. E. (2000). Emotion circuits in the brain. *Annual Review of Neuroscience*, 23, 155–184.

Leeuw, M., Goossens, M. E., Linton, S. J., Crombez, G., Boersma, K., & Vlaeyen, J. W. (2007). The fear-avoidance model of musculoskeletal pain: Current state of scientific evidence. *Journal of Behavioral Medicine*, 30(1), 77–94.

Liptan, G. (2016). *The FibroManual: A Complete Fibromyalgia Treatment Guide for You and Your Doctor.* Ballantine Books.

Lorenz, J., Minoshima, S., & Casey, K. L. (2003). Keeping pain out of mind: The role of the dorsolateral prefrontal cortex in pain modulation. *Brain*, 126(5), 1079–1091.

Louw, A., Diener, I., Butler, D. S., & Puentedura, E. J. (2011). The effect of neuroscience education on pain, disability, anxiety, and stress in chronic musculoskeletal pain. *Archives of Physical Medicine and Rehabilitation*, 92(12), 2041–2056.

Louw, A., et al. (2016). The efficacy of pain neuroscience education on musculoskeletal pain: A systematic review of the literature. *Physiotherapy Theory and Practice*, 32(5), 332–355.

Louw, A., Zimney, K., Puentedura, E. J., & Diener, I. (2016). The efficacy of pain neuroscience education on musculoskeletal pain: A systematic review of the literature. *Physiotherapy Theory and Practice*, 32(5), 332–355.

Maihöfner, C., et al. (2004). Cortical reorganization during recovery from complex regional pain syndrome. *Neurology*, 63(4), 693–701.

Maihöfner, C., Handwerker, H. O., Neundörfer, B., & Birklein, F. (2003). Patterns of cortical reorganization in complex regional pain syndrome. *Neurology*, 61(12), 1707–1715.

Malfait, F., Francomano, C., Byers, P., Belmont, J., Berglund, B., Black, J., ... & Tinkle, B. (2017). The 2017 international classification of the Ehlers-Danlos syndromes. *American Journal of Medical Genetics Part C: Seminars in Medical Genetics*, 175(1), 8–26.

Marinus, J., Moseley, G. L., Birklein, F., Baron, R., Maihöfner, C., Kingery, W. S., & van Hilten, J. J. (2011). Clinical features and pathophysiology of complex regional pain syndrome. *Lancet Neurology*, 10(7), 637–648.

Martínez-Lavín, M., Hermosillo, A. G., Rosas, M., & Soto, M. E. (1998). Circadian studies of autonomic nervous balance in patients with fibromyalgia: A heart rate variability analysis. *Arthritis & Rheumatism*, 41(11), 1966–1971.

McCracken, L. M., & Vowles, K. E. (2014). Acceptance and Commitment Therapy and mindfulness for chronic pain: Model, process, and progress. *American Psychologist*, 69(2), 178–187.

McEwen, B. S. (2006). Sleep deprivation as a neurobiologic and physiologic stressor: Allostasis and allostatic load. *Sleep*, 29(9), 1149–1155.

McEwen, B. S. (2007). Physiology and neurobiology of stress and adaptation: Central role of the brain. *Physiological Reviews*, 87(3), 873–904.

McEwen, B. S., & Kalia, M. (2010). The role of corticosteroids and stress in chronic pain conditions. *Metabolism*, 59, S9–S15.

Melzack, R., & Wall, P. D. (1965). Pain mechanisms: A new theory. *Science*, 150(3699), 971–979.

Mendell, L. M. (2014). Constructing and deconstructing the gate theory of pain. *Pain*, 155(2), 210–216.

Merzenich, M. M., & Jenkins, W. M. (1990). Reorganization of cortical representations of the hand following alterations of skin inputs. *Brain Research*, 525(2), 325–331.

Morris, G., et al. (2016). Myalgic encephalomyelitis or chronic fatigue syndrome: How could the illness develop? *Metabolic Brain Disease*, 31(3), 385–415.

Moseley, G. L. (2003). A pain neuromatrix approach to patients with chronic pain. *Manual Therapy*, 8(3), 130–140.

Moseley, G. L. (2004). Evidence for a direct relationship between cognitive and physical change during an education intervention in chronic pain. *Pain*, 109(1–2), 37–45.

Moseley, G. L. (2004). Evidence for a direct relationship between cognitive and physical change during an education intervention in chronic low back pain patients. *Pain*, 108(1–2), 192–198.

Moseley, G. L. (2006). Graded motor imagery for pathologic pain: A randomized controlled trial. *Neurology*, 67(12), 2129–2134.

Moseley, G. L., & Butler, D. S. (2015). Fifteen years of explaining pain: The past, present, and future. *Journal of Pain*, 16(9), 807–813.

Moseley, G. L., & Flor, H. (2012). Targeting cortical representations in the treatment of chronic pain: A review. *Neurorehabilitation and Neural Repair*, 26(6), 646–652.

Moseley, G. L., & Vlaeyen, J. W. (2015). Beyond nociception: The imprecision hypothesis of chronic pain. *Pain*, 156(1), 35–38.

Myers, K. M., & Davis, M. (2007). Mechanisms of fear extinction. *Neuron*, 56(5), 829–844.

Nakatomi, Y., et al. (2014). Neuroinflammation in patients with chronic fatigue syndrome/myalgic encephalomyelitis. *Journal of Nuclear Medicine*, 55(6), 945–950.

National Center for Complementary and Integrative Health (NCCIH). (2021). *Massage Therapy for Health Purposes: What You Need To Know*. U.S. Department of Health and Human Services.

Neff, K. D. (2003). Self-compassion: An alternative conceptualization of a healthy attitude toward oneself. *Self and Identity*, 2(2), 85–101.

Nijs, J., Leysen, L., Vanlauwe, J., Logghe, T., Ickmans, K., Polli, A., Malfliet, A., Coppieters, I., & Huysmans, E. (2019). Treatment of central sensitization in patients with chronic pain: Time for change? *Expert Opinion on Pharmacotherapy*, 20(16), 1961–1970.

Nijs, J., Meeus, M., Versijpt, J., Moens, M., Bos, I., Knaepen, K., & Meeusen, R. (2015). Brain-derived neurotrophic factor as a driving force behind neuroplasticity in neuropathic and central sensitization pain: A new therapeutic target? *Expert Opinion on Therapeutic Targets*, 19(4), 565–576.

Nijs, J., Paul van Wilgen, C., Van Oosterwijck, J., van Ittersum, M., & Meeus, M. (2011). How to explain central sensitization to patients with 'unexplained' chronic musculoskeletal pain: Practice guidelines. *Manual Therapy*, 16(5), 413–418.

Nijs, J., Van Houdenhove, B., & Oostendorp, R. A. (2010). Recognition of central sensitization in patients with musculoskeletal pain: Application of pain neurophysiology in manual therapy practice. *Manual Therapy*, 15(2), 135–141.

Nijs, J., Van Oosterwijck, J., De Hertogh, W., & Meeus, M. (2010). Scientific insights into chronic widespread pain and fatigue: The role of central sensitization and stress. *Current Rheumatology Reviews*, 6(3), 182–187.

Nijs, J., et al. (2015). Sleep disturbances and severe stress as glial activators: Implications for chronic pain. *Expert Review of Neurotherapeutics*, 15(5), 385–392.

Noble, D. J., & Hochman, S. (2019). Hypothesis: Oxygen and the autonomic nervous system—The oxygen–vagal theory. *Frontiers in Neuroscience*, 13, 454.

Norrholm, S. D., et al. (2011). Fear extinction in traumatized civilians with posttraumatic stress disorder. *Biological Psychiatry*, 69(6), 556–563.

Oaklander, A. L., Herzog, Z. D., Downs, H. M., & Klein, M. M. (2013). Objective evidence that small-fiber polyneuropathy underlies some illnesses currently labeled as fibromyalgia. *Pain*, 154(11), 2310–2316.

Okamoto-Mizuno, K., & Mizuno, K. (2012). Effects of thermal environment on sleep and circadian rhythm. *Journal of Physiological Anthropology*, 31(1), 14.

Ossipov, M. H., Dussor, G. O., & Porreca, F. (2010). Central modulation of pain. *Journal of Clinical Investigation*, 120(11), 3779–3787.

Palmer, S., Bailey, S., Barker, L., Barney, L., & Elliott, A. (2014). The effectiveness of therapeutic exercise for joint hypermobility syndrome: A systematic review. *Physiotherapy*, 100(3), 220–227.

Paulus, M. P., & Stein, M. B. (2010). Interoception in anxiety and depression. *Brain Structure and Function*, 214(5-6), 451–463.

Penfield, W., & Boldrey, E. (1937). Somatic motor and sensory representation in the cerebral cortex of man as studied by electrical stimulation. *Brain*, 60(4), 389–443.

Pincus, T., & McCracken, L. M. (2013). Psychological factors and treatment opportunities in low back pain. *Best Practice & Research Clinical Rheumatology*, 27(5), 625–635.

Popkin, B. M., et al. (2010). Water, hydration, and health. *Nutrition Reviews*, 68(8), 439–458.

Porges, S. W. (2011). *The Polyvagal Theory: Neurophysiological Foundations of Emotions, Attachment, Communication, and Self-regulation*. W. W. Norton & Company.

Proal, A. D., & Marshall, T. G. (2018). Myalgic encephalomyelitis/chronic fatigue syndrome in the era of the human microbiome. *Microbiome*, 6, 120.

Proske, U., & Gandevia, S. C. (2012). The proprioceptive senses: Their roles in signaling body shape, body position and movement, and muscle force. *Physiological Reviews*, 92(4), 1651–1697.

Pujol, J., López-Solà, M., Ortiz, H., et al. (2009). Mapping brain response to pain in fibromyalgia patients using temporal analysis of fMRI. *PLOS ONE*, 4(4), e5224.

Qaseem, A., et al. (2017). Noninvasive treatments for acute, subacute, and chronic low back pain: A clinical practice guideline from the American College of Physicians. *Annals of Internal Medicine*, 166(7), 514–530.

Rainville, P., Duncan, G. H., Price, D. D., Carrier, B., & Bushnell, M. C. (1997). Pain affect encoded in human anterior cingulate but not somatosensory cortex. *Science*, 277(5328), 968–971.

Raj, S. R. (2013). Postural tachycardia syndrome (POTS). *Circulation*, 127(23), 2336–2342.

Ramachandran, V. S., & Altschuler, E. L. (2009). The use of visual feedback, in particular mirror visual feedback, in restoring brain function. *Brain*, 132(7), 1693–1710.

Roehrs, T., Hyde, M., Blaisdell, B., Greenwald, M., & Roth, T. (2006). Sleep loss and REM sleep loss are hyperalgesic. *Sleep*, 29(2), 145–151.

Roehrs, T., & Roth, T. (2005). Sleep and pain: Interaction of two vital functions. *Seminars in Neurology*, 25(1), 106–116.

Ruscio, A. M., & Borkovec, T. D. (2004). Experience and appraisal of worry among high worriers with and without generalized anxiety disorder. *Behaviour Research and Therapy*, 42(12), 1469–1482.

Sack, R. L., Auckley, D., Auger, R. R., Carskadon, M. A., Wright, K. P., Vitiello, M. V., Zhdanova, I. V., & The Standards of Practice Committee of the American Academy of Sleep Medicine. (2007). Circadian rhythm sleep disorders: Part II, advanced sleep phase disorder and delayed sleep phase disorder. *Sleep*, 30(11), 1484–1501.

Sandkühler, J. (2009). Models and mechanisms of hyperalgesia and allodynia. *Physiological Reviews*, 89(2), 707–758.

Sapolsky, R. M. (2004). *Why Zebras Don't Get Ulcers* (3rd ed.). Holt Paperbacks.

Sarlani, E., & Greenspan, J. D. (2005). Why look in the brain for answers to temporomandibular disorder pain? *Cells Tissues Organs*, 180(1), 69–75.

Scheper, M. C., Nicholson, L. L., & Engelbert, R. H. (2017). Chronic pain in hypermobility syndrome and Ehlers–Danlos syndrome—Hypermobility type: It is a challenge. *Journal of Pain Research*, 10, 1169–1178.

Scheper, M. C., Rombaut, L., de Vries, J. E., De Wandele, I., van der Esch, M., Visser, B., ... & Engelbert, R. H. (2017). The association between muscle strength and activity limitations in patients with the hypermobility type of Ehlers-Danlos syndrome: The impact of proprioception. *Disability and Rehabilitation*, 39(14), 1391–1397.

Shah, J. P., et al. (2015). Myofascial trigger points then and now: A historical and scientific perspective. *PM&R*, 7(7), 746–761.

Simons, D. G., Travell, J. G., & Simons, L. S. (1999). *Travell & Simons' Myofascial Pain and Dysfunction: The*

Trigger Point Manual (2nd ed.). Lippincott Williams & Wilkins.

Simons, D. G., Travell, J. G., & Simons, L. S. (1999). *Travell & Simons' Myofascial Pain and Dysfunction: The Trigger Point Manual* (2nd ed.). Williams & Wilkins.

Skeldon, A. C., Phillips, A. J., & Dijk, D. J. (2017). The effects of self-selected light-dark cycles and social constraints on human sleep and circadian timing: A modeling approach. *Scientific Reports*, 7, 45158.

Smith, M. T., & Haythornthwaite, J. A. (2004). How do sleep disturbance and chronic pain inter-relate? Insights from the longitudinal and cognitive-behavioral clinical trials literature. *Sleep Medicine Reviews*, 8(2), 119–132.

Squire, L. R., & Zola, S. M. (1996). Structure and function of declarative and nondeclarative memory systems. *Proceedings of the National Academy of Sciences*, 93(24), 13515–13522.

Staud, R., Vierck, C. J., Cannon, R. L., Mauderli, A. P., & Price, D. D. (2001). Abnormal sensitization and temporal summation of second pain (wind-up) in patients with fibromyalgia syndrome. *Pain*, 91(1–2), 165–175.

Stewart, J. M., et al. (2012). Mechanisms of sympathetic regulation in orthostatic intolerance. *Journal of Applied Physiology*, 113(10), 1659–1668.

Sturgeon, J. A., & Zautra, A. J. (2016). Social pain and physical pain: Shared paths to resilience. *Pain Management*, 6(1), 63–74.

Sullivan, M. J., Bishop, S. R., & Pivik, J. (1995). The Pain Catastrophizing Scale: Development and validation. *Psychological Assessment*, 7(4), 524–532.

Sullivan, M. J., Thorn, B., Haythornthwaite, J. A., Keefe, F., Martin, M., Bradley, L. A., & Lefebvre, J. C. (2001). Theoretical perspectives on the relation between catastrophizing and pain. *The Clinical Journal of Pain*, 17(1), 52–64.

Tang, N. K., Goodchild, C. E., Sanborn, A. N., Howard, J., & Salkovskis, P. M. (2012). Deciphering the temporal link between pain and sleep in a heterogeneous chronic pain patient sample: A multilevel daily process study. *Sleep*, 35(5), 675–687.

Theoharides, T. C., Stewart, J. M., Hatziagelaki, E., & Kolaitis, G. (2015). Brain "fog," inflammation and obesity: Key aspects of neuropsychiatric disorders improved by luteolin. *Frontiers in Neuroscience*, 9, 225.

Tracey, I., & Mantyh, P. W. (2007). The cerebral signature for pain perception and its modulation. *Neuron*, 55(3), 377–391.

Trauer, J. M., Qian, M. Y., Doyle, J. S., Rajaratnam, S. M., & Cunnington, D. (2015). Cognitive behavioral therapy for chronic insomnia: A systematic review and meta-analysis. *Annals of Internal Medicine*, 163(3), 191–204.

Uceyler, N., Eberle, T., Rolke, R., Birklein, F., & Sommer, C. (2007). Differential expression patterns of cytokines in complex regional pain syndrome. *Pain*, 132(1-2), 195–205.

van der Kolk, B. A. (2014). *The Body Keeps the Score: Brain, Mind, and Body in the Healing of Trauma*. Viking.

Van Cauter, E., & Plat, L. (1996). Physiology of growth hormone secretion during sleep. *Journal of Pediatrics*, 128(5 Pt 2), S32–S37.

Vickhoff, B., et al. (2013). Music structure determines heart rate variability of singers. *Frontiers in Psychology*, 4, 334.

Vlaeyen, J. W., de Jong, J., Geilen, M., Heuts, P. H., & van Breukelen, G. (2001). Graded exposure in vivo in the treatment of pain-related fear: A replicated single-case experimental design in four patients with chronic low back pain. *Behaviour Research and Therapy*, 39(2), 151–166.

Vlaeyen, J. W., & Linton, S. J. (2000). Fear-avoidance and its consequences in chronic musculoskeletal pain: A state of the art. *Pain*, 85(3), 317–332.

Vlaeyen, J. W., & Linton, S. J. (2012). Fear-avoidance model of chronic musculoskeletal pain: 12 years on. *Pain*, 153(6), 1144–1147.

Vlaeyen, J. W. S., & Linton, S. J. (2012). Fear-avoidance model of chronic musculoskeletal pain: 12 years on. *Pain*, 153(6), 1144–1147.

Walker, M. P. (2009). The role of sleep in cognition and emotion. *Annals of the New York Academy of Sciences*, 1156(1), 168–197.

West, C., Stewart, L., Foster, K., & Usher, K. (2012). The meaning of chronic pain: A qualitative meta-synthesis. *International Journal of Nursing Studies*, 49(6), 698–710.

Wiech, K., & Tracey, I. (2013). Pain, decisions, and actions: A motivational perspective. *Frontiers in Neuroscience*, 7, 46.

Williams, A. C. D. C., Fisher, E., Hearn, L., & Eccleston, C. (2020). Psychological therapies for the management of chronic pain (excluding headache) in adults. *Cochrane Database of Systematic Reviews*, 8, CD007407.

Woolf, C. J. (2011). Central sensitization: Implications for the diagnosis and treatment of pain. *Pain*, 152(3 Suppl), S2–S15.

Woolf, C. J., & Ma, Q. (2007). Nociceptors—noxious stimulus detectors. *Neuron*, 55(3), 353–364.

Woolf, C. J., & Salter, M. W. (2000). Neuronal plasticity: Increasing the gain in pain. *Science*, 288(5472), 1765–1769.

Yunus, M. B. (2007). Fibromyalgia and overlapping disorders: The unifying concept of central sensitivity syndromes. *Seminars in Arthritis and Rheumatism*, 36(6), 339–356.

Yunus, M. B. (2007). Role of central sensitization in symptoms of fibromyalgia. *The American Journal of Medicine*, 120(Suppl 1), S3–S13.

Zaccaro, A., Piarulli, A., Laurino, M., Garbella, E., Menicucci, D., Neri, B., & Gemignani, A. (2018). How breath-control can change your life: A systematic review on psycho-physiological correlates of slow breathing. *Frontiers in Human Neuroscience*, 12, 353.

Zeidan, F., Adler-Neal, A. L., Wells, R. E., Stagnaro, E., May, L. M., Eisenach, J. C., McHaffie, J. G., & Coghill, R. C. (2016). Mindfulness-meditation-based pain relief is not mediated by endogenous opioids. *The Journal of Neuroscience*, 36(11), 3391–3397.

About the Author

Jerry has spent more than two decades working at the intersection of performance and pain management. He is a licensed massage therapist specializing in orthopedic, neuromuscular, and myoskeletal alignment work, a personal trainer with a background in strength and conditioning and corrective exercise, and a wellness coach who turns every session into a coaching conversation. Over the years he has worked with weekend warriors, CrossFit athletes, professional athletes, and Olympic competitors. Even so, the core of his practice has always been the same: helping people in pain make sense of what is happening in their bodies.

Early in his career, Jerry became known in his local community for working with chronic pain cases that never fit neatly into diagnostic boxes. Physicians and physical therapists began referring patients with complex conditions ranging from persistent injuries to fibromyalgia, Ehlers-Danlos Syndrome, CRPS, and other disorders that resisted easy explanation.

Jerry became consumed with the question beneath the question: not only how to treat pain, but why it behaves the way it does. That drive led to years of studying pain neuroscience and movement mechanics. It also fueled a growing frustration with the gaps in how pain is explained to patients, to providers, and even within the research itself.

This book is an attempt to do in writing what Jerry has spent two decades doing in practice: translating complex pain science into something useful, validating lived experience without false promises, and offering a framework that finally makes sense of why chronic pain behaves the way it does. It is not a cure. It is a map. And for people who have been lost in the system, a map is often the most valuable thing they can get.

Jerry lives in Lafayette, Louisiana, and continues to work with clients navigating chronic pain and athletic performance.

www.ingramcontent.com/pod-product-compliance
Lightning Source LLC
LaVergne TN
LVHW041737060526
838201LV00046B/838